Solving the Frontline Crisis in Long-term Care

**A PRACTICAL GUIDE
TO FINDING AND KEEPING
QUALITY NURSING ASSISTANTS**

— Dr. Karl Pillemer —

A SPECIAL REPORT FROM FRONTLINE PUBLISHING CORP.,
PUBLISHERS OF **NURSING ASSISTANT MONTHLY**

ISBN 0-9653629-0-6

Please Note: Advice given in this book is general. Readers should consult professional counsel for specific legal, ethical, or clinical questions.

SPECIAL DISCOUNTS

Solving the Frontline Crisis in Long-term Care is available at special discounts for bulk purchases. For details, contact the General Manager, Frontline Publishing.

FRONTLINE PUBLISHING

Frontline Publishing is the publisher of **Nursing Assistant Monthly**, an ongoing continuing education program designed specifically for nursing assistants in long-term care. Based on more than ten years of research by Cornell gerontologist Dr. Karl Pillemer, the program is designed to help facilities train, develop and retain frontline staff. A complete listing of Nursing Assistant Monthly is found in Appendix 3 in the back of this book along with a coupon for a free sample. For more information, contact:

Frontline Publishing Corporation
17 Herbert Street, PO Box 441002
Somerville, MA 02144
Telephone: 1-800-348-0605
Fax: 1-617-625-7446
Web: www.frontlinepub.com

This book is dedicated to the memory of Vivienne Wisdom, former Executive Director of the New Hampshire Health Care Association, and national leader in efforts to promote quality nursing home care. Vivienne's enthusiasm and encouragement for my interest in improving the work life of frontline staff was a continual inspiration to me.

I would also like to thank the main characters in the story you are about to read: the nursing assistants. I would like to acknowledge not only the hundreds of frontline workers who have participated in our studies, but everyone who takes on the challenging but rewarding work of caring for our frail older citizens. This book is for you.

TABLE OF CONTENTS

NOTE TO THE READER

We have done our best to make it as easy as possible for you to follow up on recommendations on this report. Therefore, the report contains three appendices. The first appendix offers a summary list of all the various ideas presented in this report. The second appendix contains works cited in each chapter, as well as other sources for further information. The third tells you how to get more information on programs cited. Since addresses and telephone numbers sometimes change, if you have difficulty finding any of the resources mentioned, feel free to contact us at the number below. Any other comments or questions about the report are also appreciated.

A number of the quotes from individuals in this report come from interviews published in Nursing Assistant Monthly. For the complete interview, contact us at Frontline Publishing (800-348-0605).

ACKNOWLEDGEMENTS

This book would never have come into being without the commitment of Frontline Publishing, and especially Martin Schumacher, Richard Hoffman, Philip Johnson, and Doug Adams. I am also grateful to the many facilities and individuals who are involved in the Nursing Assistant Monthly program, and to members of our advisory board; it is through my discussions and involvement with them that the idea for this book came about. Thanks are also due to the individuals who reviewed and commented on earlier drafts of this book: Reg Carter, Elise Nakhnikian, Richard Peck, and Carol Tschop.

ABOUT THE AUTHOR

Karl Pillemer, Ph.D., an internationally known geron-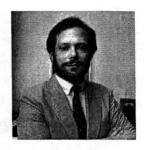
tologist and sociologist, is Associate Professor at
Cornell University and Director of the Cornell Applied
Gerontology Research Institute.

Widely sought after as a speaker, Dr. Pillemer has co-
authored or edited three books, and published over 50
academic articles. Much of his research has been devoted to the development
of model projects for nursing homes. He is a co-founder and the Executive
Editor of Nursing Assistant Monthly, an ongoing professional development and
education program for frontline staff in long-term care.

FOREWORD

Consistency is the heart of quality care in a nursing home. Our elderly want and deserve to be cared for by staff who know them as people and respect their individual needs and preferences. Indeed, many would say that such an individual approach is the very definition of quality care. It follows that the best investment in quality for any nursing facility is a firm commitment to lowering staff turnover.

The book you are holding in your hand offers numerous solutions to the turnover problem. It will change the way you think about your frontline staff. It will offer you new ways to find and train these caregivers. It will help you build morale and create loyalty. With *Solving the Front-line Crisis in Long-term Care* we have, at last, a thorough and thoughtful discussion of the entire complex issue of recruitment and retention, along with a goldmine of "best practices" from innovative providers across the country. Based on over a decade of research into the lives of frontline caregiving staff, this book will help you to understand what's at the root of your particular turnover problem, and enable you to create a strategy clearly linked to the real issues you face.

Dr. Pillemer's in-depth understanding of the world of the nursing assistant, both on and off the job, provides us with valuable information about these essential employees and their experience, hopes, and dreams. Taking a simple, direct approach, Dr. Pillemer leads us from a survey of the problem to new understandings we can build upon in fashioning a loyal and stable frontline staff for the future. In its clarity, scope, and usefulness, this book has the potential to free the long-term care industry from the demoralizing problem of turnover, so destructive to all our best efforts to provide quality care.

As Director of the Applied Gerontology Research Institute at Cornell University, and as Executive Editor of Nursing Assistant Monthly, a program designed to reduce turnover by developing the interpersonal and psychosocial skills of CNAs, Dr. Pillemer remains intimately aware of the day-to-day operations of nursing homes throughout the country. His experienced approach to the problems of providers makes *Solving the Frontline Crisis in Long-term Care* an invaluable resource for administrators, human resource managers, directors of nursing, staff developers, and others involved in finding and keeping the kind of caregivers our elderly deserve.

Reginald Carter, Ph.D.
Executive Vice President
Health Care Association of Michigan

Solving the Frontline Crisis
in Long-term Care

CHAPTER ONE

Introduction: a Time to Act

When I started out ten years ago to study frontline staff in nursing homes, little did I realize how much of a passion (some of my colleagues would say an obsession!) this topic would become for me.

I still remember the first focus group discussion we held in 1986 with nursing assistants, over coffee and doughnuts in the under-heated conference room of a large New England nursing home. I remember the eagerness of the staff, the happiness that, finally, someone wanted to hear **their** story. I was moved by their description of the difficulties of their job, the physical stress and emotional strain, and the struggle to balance their work with pressures in their personal lives.

Most of all, I was moved by the quiet heroism I saw in these workers. Sure, they weren't perfect, and they knew it. But they were committed to providing quality care, a kind of care that goes beyond keeping people clean and fed. The kind of care that means taking the time to laugh with residents, to pray with them, to hold the hand of a dying person, or to calm the fears of an anxious family member.

Looking back on it now, as I left the nursing home that night, I was a changed person. I had worked with nursing homes for years, but that evening I had received the proverbial whack on the head. Two things seemed suddenly clear to me. I realized that nursing assistants are a tremendous **resource,** and not a **problem** to be managed. And in that moment I also knew that no matter how closely nursing homes follow regulations, no matter what new products they buy, no matter how much money they spend — none of it makes any difference without the nursing assistant.

Nursing assistants are
the key to quality care.

This truth lodged itself in my brain that night, and a decade later it is the core of our philosophy at Frontline Publishing. We have learned that when we invest in frontline staff, and when we value them, everyone benefits — nurses, administrators, families, and, most of all, the residents. After ten years, I can honestly state that I find our work more and more exciting as each day goes by. We are continually learning what **works** to maintain a caring, committed frontline staff.

In this report, I want to share some of these ideas with you. If I have done my job, then you will become as excited as we are about upgrading your frontline workforce. It takes effort, patience, and imagination, but the payoff in worker and resident satisfaction, decreased turnover, quality of care, and efficiency are well worth the effort.

Turn Frustration into Creativity

My colleagues and I at Frontline Publishing have spent much of the past two years talking to people in the nursing home industry. We've sat with executives from state long-term care associations. We've given presentations to hundreds of administrators at meetings across the country. As publishers of **Nursing Assistant Monthly,** a comprehensive continuing education program for nursing assistants, we're in touch with dozens of directors of nursing and staff development coordinators every month. We've asked the same questions over and over: What's going on with nursing assistants where you are? Can you find them? Can you keep them? What are you doing about recruitment and retention?

What we hear is **frustration.** People feel defeated and helpless. No matter where you go, in urban areas or rural communities, in all parts of the country, we hear things like this:

"I just can't find the staff I need!"

"Help — Our turnover rate is 100%!"

"It's a revolving door here with the nursing assistants: for every person I hire, someone leaves."

And we almost always hear this: "Nothing I do seems to make any difference."

The tragedy here is that this **does not have to be the case!** There are actually lots of creative solutions out there for recruitment and retention problems. Some of these solutions can be implemented **immediately.** You can read this report, put it down, and start them tomorrow (and we hope you will!). Some of the best ideas don't require a strategic plan, consultants, or a lot of staff time. All they take is someone who is willing to give a new idea a try.

Some of the other ideas contained in this report take more time and planning. A few can best be carried out in cooperation with other providers and organizations. As we will show later on, such efforts have long-term payoffs that are well worth the effort.

The best cure for the frontline blues is an **active** stance. Instead of frustration, the good news from the field is that by working creatively **now** to improve recruitment and retention of nursing assistants, your facility can place itself in a strong position for years to come.

What will this report do for you? First, it will help you to diagnose your recruitment and retention problems. It deflates some of the myths about nursing assistants, and helps you understand these workers better. You will learn to calculate turnover rates, and to understand why your staff leave.

But understanding the current situation isn't enough. So the second goal of this report is to help you decide what you should **do** about your recruitment and retention problems. For once, the news is good: our review of "best practices" from around the country has uncovered many excellent solutions, ready for you to use.

Three Cardinal Principles

By now, we hope you are eager to get into the report, and to get started solving recruitment and retention problems. Before we move on, however, we want to sum up what we've learned over the past decade into three points. It's not an exaggeration to say that if a facility consistently practices these three principles, it will have made a huge step toward building a committed frontline workforce.

1. Investigate

To win at the recruitment and retention game, your facility has to take a good, hard look at itself. You have to sit down with your staff and ask questions like this: How big is our turnover problem here? Who is leaving, and who is staying? Most important of all, **why** do staff leave? You need to **diagnose** your individual facility's recruitment and retention problems. What works somewhere else may not necessarily work for you. You need to understand your own frontline staff — this is one case where knowledge really **is** power!

2. Innovate

Guess what? **Everybody wants your frontline employees.** It's true: every restaurant, every hotel, every hospital, and of course every other nursing home wants your good frontline staff. The pool of frontline workers is shrinking, and you've got to compete to get the staff you need.

Frankly, it is amazing to us how few nursing homes have realized the truth of this critical fact. All too many facilities just assume that, somehow, frontline workers will continue to trickle in through the door. It's just not true. It will get harder and harder to maintain a competent frontline work force in the current market.

So this is no time to stand on the sidelines; other employers will snap up the pool of qualified frontline employees. You **must** have an active stance. Nursing homes should be ready to make both short-term innovations to relieve their immediate staffing problems, as well as developing one-, two-, and even five- or ten-year strategies for developing the workforce they need.

After researching and diagnosing your recruitment and retention problems, try some new approaches. If they don't work, try something else. Or somebody else will!

3. Respect

If we have learned one thing from talking to hundreds of nursing assistants, it's that the key to retaining them is **respect**. All too often, supervisors and administrators see nursing assistants as replaceable, unskilled labor. And nothing could be further from the truth!

As we will show later on in this report, nursing assistants are usually deeply committed, highly motivated individuals, who are asked to perform tasks that are very psychologically demanding. They leave because they feel that neither they nor their work are respected. Recognizing that nursing assistants are the key to quality care, and treating them as such, are the first important steps you can take to solve your frontline staffing problems.

If you are interested enough in your nursing assistants to be reading this report, I'll bet you have already made a start in these three areas. As I said earlier, knowledge is power. In the next two chapters, we'll focus on background knowledge about the current situation that will help you be a winner at recruitment and retention.

CHAPTER TWO

The Demographic Wake-up Call

We've got a problem. You'll notice that I said "we" and not "you." That's because all of us — the entire long-term care system, in fact — is on the edge of a crisis in frontline staffing.

When my colleagues and I have talked to administrators, we've found that they (like most of us) tend to personalize their problems. They see their difficulties attracting and keeping staff as a personal failure. So it may help to know that when it comes to building a good frontline nursing home workforce, **everyone** is being hurt by national trends that influence the labor conditions for paraprofessionals.

"Crisis" is an overused term these days. But based on the trends, I do not think it is an exaggeration to say that we are entering into a crisis situation regarding nursing assistants. To put it bluntly: You may think you are having a difficult time recruiting and retaining nursing assistants now, but if we don't respond to the challenges of the current situation, "you ain't seen nothin' yet!"

This does not mean that facilities should despair, but rather that they should **prepare.** Nursing homes that listen to the demographic wake-up call will place themselves in a much stronger position when the crunch hits.

Why is the demographic alarm clock ringing? Three major factors will have the biggest impact.

TREND NUMBER 1:

The dramatic growth in the elderly population is placing new demands on the long-term care system.

You've heard this so many times, you probably considered skipping this one. But have you really thought about what it means in terms of frontline staff?

What's going to happen? By the year 2030, the population age 65 and over in the U.S. is expected to double, and the number of persons 85 and over will increase by five times the current number, from 3.2 million in 1990 to more than 15 million. Further, the number of elderly people living in the community who need long-term care is expected to grow from seven million to nearly 14 million.

But it's not going to take 35 years for us to start feeling the impact of the aging of our society. Every year, the elderly population grows, and with that growth come increased numbers of elderly persons with severe physical and mental disabilities, who need long-term care. And who will care for them? Nursing assistants.

Over the next decades, then, we will need hundreds of thousands of new frontline workers, workers who are willing to take on a very stressful and demanding job. In fact, both *Time Magazine* and the *Wall Street Journal* have identified nursing assistants as one of the fastest-growing occupations over the next decade.

Estimates vary about how many new nursing assistants will be needed in the next ten years. Of course, this depends on many things, including whether states carry out moratoriums on the construction of long-term care beds. The U.S. Bureau of Labor Statistics estimates that we will need nearly **600,000** new nursing assistants by early in the next decade. A question on everyone's mind should be: Where are these workers going to come from?

TREND NUMBER 2:

The nursing home population is becoming older, sicker, frailer, and more complicated to care for.

The emphasis on transferring elderly people from acute to long-term care settings as quickly as possible has resulted from the Medicare prospective payment system and from DRGs. This trend toward earlier discharge means that more residents have acute illnesses from which they have not completely recovered. One sign of this trend is that nursing homes are now using more complicated technologies that earlier were used only in hospitals.

The burden of care for this increasingly impaired population will fall on the nursing assistants. Although nursing assistants are less than one half of all nursing home personnel, it is estimated that they provide close to 90% of all the care residents receive.

As one nursing assistant told us: "Things have changed so much over the past ten years. We used to be able to sit and talk, or do someone's hair, or even play cards for a little while. And the residents were not so bad off, and they could tell us that they appreciated what we did. It's not like that anymore."

By every account, this state of affairs has resulted in a dramatic increase in the workload for nursing assistants in nursing homes. A recent survey of nursing homes shows that more than 90% reported that their residents are more likely now to require more hours of care than five years ago. They also reported that their residents are sicker than ever before.

Further, many nursing homes are moving into the post-acute and sub-acute markets, which characteristically involve an even more intensive level of care and expertise from staff. And in some facilities, the resident population is becoming more complex, as nursing homes make room for AIDS patients, younger disabled clients, or the mentally ill.

TREND NUMBER 3:

The labor force won't respond by itself to the need for more frontline long-term care workers.

In general, the labor force as a whole is growing much more slowly than the population is growing older. And this is especially so when we look at potential long-term care workers. The number of young adults — who make up a large percentage of nursing assistants — is decreasing in relation to the elderly population. Between 1990 and 2020, the number of people over 50 will increase by 74% while those under 50, their potential caregivers, will increase by only one percent. Further, restrictions on immigration have been enacted, which will probably get even stronger in the future. This is a special problem in many areas, where recent immigrants make up a sizable part of the frontline nursing home workforce. These two trends alone will result in a decreased supply of new workers.

So, staff shortages are likely to plague nursing homes for years to come. The Massachusetts Extended Care Federation learned just that when they conducted a study of employee shortages in its facilities. Of the 227 facilities surveyed, more than 90% of the facilities said they were suffering from shortages of nursing assistants, with three-quarters saying the problem was moderate or severe. The pool of applicants, they said, was shrinking, and those people who did apply had poor job histories and habits, and little experience with the elderly and disabled.

In a follow-up study, the Federation surveyed 95 facilities in depth. According to that survey, 44% of these facilities were short-staffed the previous day. On the 3-11 shift, for example, there was a 23% shortage of staff. From everything we've heard, the problem is probably as bad — or worse — in other states.

Okay, there it is: the bad news. Maybe you knew all this already. Possibly your response has been to throw up your hands, decide to do your best, and take the worst when it comes, living one day (or one nursing assistant vacancy) at a time.

Or maybe your response was different (and I hope it was). Perhaps you see these trends not just as challenges, but as opportunities. Based on our study of best practices around the country, we would definitely encourage this point of view. Your facility can master this problem, with a little planning and effort.

A good first step is taking an in-depth look at nursing assistants. To do that, we need to explode some myths about who nursing assistants are.

CHAPTER THREE

Six Myths about Nursing Assistants

When I talk to groups of administrators about nursing assistants, I sometimes surprise them with the question: "Would **you** like to be a nursing assistant?" There is usually some hemming and hawing, and a little nervous laughter. Then the brave ones say out loud what the others are thinking: "No thanks!"

So let's get this truth out in the open: most of us professionals who work with nursing assistants — hiring them, supervising them (or in my case, studying them) — wouldn't want to **be** one of them. Many of us have negative stereotypes about the job that keep us from understanding the nursing assistants and their work experience.

There is another barrier to understanding the work life of nursing assistants. One thing that decades of sociological research have taught us is that there isn't just one way of life in a nursing home, one way of looking at things. Sociologist Jaber Gubrium made this clear when he discovered that the various groups in the nursing home — administrators, nurses, nursing assistants, and residents — live in what he termed different "worlds."

Each person's job in the nursing home shapes his or her view of life there. Different groups have different goals, and see the nursing home "world" differently. This means that administrators and nursing supervisors have to make a special effort to see the world as the nursing assistant sees it. A little like an anthropologist, they have to get rid of their stereotypes, and understand what nursing assistants are **really** like.

Some administrators, of course, have a good understanding of nursing assistants. Take Dr. Mark Jerstad, President and CEO of the Evangelical Lutheran Good Samaritan Society, which has over 200 nursing homes. Rather than just talk to nursing assistants, he decided to **become** one! He went through the training program and became a CNA. In his words, "Becoming a CNA is a gift. It has shaped me. It has influenced my thinking in lots of important ways." All executives in the organization must now spend one day each year working side-by-side with a CNA.

But in our discussions throughout the country, we have found that myths about CNAs tend to be more common than this kind of first-hand knowledge. In this chapter, we'd like to give you a perspective on the world of the nursing assistant, by pointing out some myths about nursing assistants that can keep administrators and supervisors from truly understanding them.

MYTH NUMBER 1:

Nursing assistants are "unskilled" labor.

Unskilled labor means workers who are easily replaceable because they do not have specialized knowledge about their jobs. Management consultant Harvey Gittler puts the lie to this myth by suggesting that we imagine what would happen if all of the nursing assistants in a facility were to quit over the weekend. Their knowledge of the residents and their needs, to say nothing of resident care skills and facility policies, would require months or years to replace.

In fact, nursing assistants are routinely put into situations that require **unusually** sophisticated interpersonal and communication skills. They are called upon to manage conflict, make ethical decisions, understand complex developmental and psychological changes, grieve and help others to grieve, and support other members of the caregiving team.

Consider these examples from what could be a typical nursing assistant's day:

- An angry family member demands an explanation for a resident's missing dress.

- A favorite resident dies.

- A resident on a restricted diet begs for just one piece of candy.

- A 95-year-old resident begins to weep and cries out for her mother.

- Two residents have a violent argument.

- A resident makes offensive, lewd suggestions.

- A demented resident becomes physically aggressive on the elevator.

Unfortunately, because the nursing assistants are often considered "unskilled," they are rarely given the kinds of training needed to address complex psychosocial problems. In many cases, we are failing to provide these all-important caregivers with the tools and resources they need to cope with such situations.

MYTH NUMBER 2:

All in all, being a nursing assistant is a pretty bad job.

Many people have negative impressions of nursing homes. If truth were told, some administrators and supervisors share this negative image of nursing assistants' work. They feel like it is a job they would not want to do.

Therefore, we can easily lose sight of the fact that nursing homes provide employment **advantages** for many types of workers: people who are young and lack experience, new immigrants, women re-entering the labor force, senior citizens interested in part-time work after retirement, and a number of others.

Have you seen the film *Hoop Dreams*? For anyone interested in nursing assistants, one scene is worth the price of admission. *Hoop Dreams* is an award-winning documentary about the lives of two talented, but poor, African-American basketball players, that follows them and their families from high school through college. The mother of one of these kids has struggled with poverty in the inner city all her life, and is very discouraged.

But then she enters a CNA training program. She succeeds, graduates at the top of her class, and lands a job. The scene that chokes audiences up is this woman's joy at passing the CNA exam. Dressed in her white uniform, tears streaming down her face, she says something like: "I never thought I'd amount to anything. And look at me now!"

The moral here is: that there are lots of people who see (or who **could** see, given the right information) being a nursing assistant as a **great** job.

It's not just Hollywood that tells us this truth; so does research. Dianne Brannon and her colleagues at the Pennsylvania State University looked at how nursing assistants rate their jobs. She found that nursing homes can market themselves to employees as places that offer opportunities to perform meaningful, caring work. They note that while the menial aspects of some tasks can't be eliminated, it is possible to present them as part of a larger caregiving role that has satisfying qualities not available in other types of work.

Their research shows that nursing homes typically **undersell** the nursing assistant job, and the quality of nursing homes as a setting in which to work — especially in comparison to the other types of jobs that are available at the same level.

Another very appealing aspect of being a nursing assistant is that it is seen as an attractive job in the health care sector. Nursing assistants themselves often view the job as an important position in the health care field. They see it as a position of responsibility. Further — and this is very important to some people — our research found that a factor in choosing the job is that nursing homes are viewed as safe and clean environments in which to work. Compared to a fast-food restaurant, or a factory, this is a major plus to many people.

It is also seen as a **respected** job. As Genevieve Gipson, expert on nursing assistants and founder of Career Nurse Assistants Day, notes: "Nursing assistants are often perceived by their friends and family as experts on health care. Their families value what they do, and come to them for advice. This kind of attention is very validating for the nursing assistant."

Maybe it is best to let the nursing assistants speak for themselves. Rosie Farmer and Phyllis Washington are both CNAs at Hoyt Nursing Home in Saginaw, Michigan. Listen to what they say about their work:

Rosie Farmer: *"I love my job. I feel good when I'm here. I work with great people. If things on the outside aren't so good, I come in here where the people need me, and I get busy. Pretty soon I feel better. It's like I remember what's important."*

Phyllis Washington: *"My work here helps me a lot. Helping people makes me feel good. When I'm off from work for a few days, I miss it. It eases my mind. I have to tell you, when I first started this job, I thought, 'Oh boy, I'm sure not going to like this!' But after just a little while, I loved it. I have such important relationships with my residents, and even the ones I don't take care of see me in the hall and say hello and call me by my name. It's a great feeling."*

Read these quotes again. Then ask yourself if you are surprised to hear statements like these. If you are, you could benefit by taking a look at the **positive** side of nursing assistant work.

MYTH NUMBER 3:

Nursing assistants are in it for the money.

The myth here is the belief that "if they weren't working here, they'd be working in McDonald's." A pervasive belief about nursing assistants is that they select nursing home work for the money, or because no other jobs are available. People tend to think that nursing assistants would just as readily flip burgers or clean hotel rooms as work in the nursing home. And nothing could be further from the truth.

Working as a nursing assistant can clearly be very demanding. So why do people choose nursing home work over comparably-paid service jobs? Over the past ten years, my colleagues and I have devoted a lot of time to understanding why nursing assistants choose their job. Because it's here that we can find the answer to the "why not McDonald's" question.

In one of our surveys, we asked approximately 600 nursing assistants why they chose nursing home work. They rated twelve possible reasons that have been found to be important to people in selecting jobs. "Because I need the money" was the **eighth** most popular answer.

Key Reasons for Selecting Nursing Home Work

What were the most important reasons for selecting nursing home work? Interestingly, they were the same reasons that many **professionals** choose their jobs. Three were clustered at the top, with most of the nursing assistants giving them the highest rating:

- It gives me an opportunity to help others (96%).

- It makes me feel meaningful (93%).

- It is useful to society (84%).

In my view, this is great news. I would call these reasons "other-centered." That is, a major motivator for nursing assistants is the chance to contribute, to do something for others, to gain a sense of meaning. You may think this sounds idealistic, or that I can't be talking about your nursing assistants. But believe me — every study we have conducted shows the same thing — a huge motivator for nursing assistants is the desire for meaningful, helping work.

After these "big three" reasons comes a second set, that reflects more of a self-interested motivation. But again, we see the kind of motivation any employer would love. The next three most important reasons, rated high by the nursing assistants, have to do with the job itself. These are:

- It offers a lot of contact with others (81%).

- It is an interesting job (73%).

- It gives me the chance to do responsible tasks (72%).

Do you see a trend here? Again, these are the same kinds of motivations many professionals cite. Indeed, it would be hard to find fast-food employees who could say that they chose their jobs for these kinds of reasons: their jobs just don't offer such intangible benefits.

Other more "materialistic" reasons — like needing the money or job security — fell a long way below the top six.

I don't know how you react to this information, but when I first looked over my computer print-outs, my jaw dropped. I had fully expected that, like frontline workers in many industries, money, job security, and other "bread-and-butter" issues would be on top. As I saw our results confirmed in study after study, I realized we had a special group of workers here.

One more point. In our focus group discussions with nursing assistants, we have asked them: "If you suddenly lost your job and no other nursing home work were available, what kind of work would you do?" Almost all of the respondents said that they would seek out other human service work, such as home health care or child care. Very few suggested that they would work in the hospitality, restaurant, or related industries. They are committed to helping people.

The point is not just to pat ourselves on the back that we have such great employees. This knowledge about motivation is something we can **use.** It gives nursing homes a "hook" to attract good employees that other front-line employers don't have. And by working to fulfill these motivations for seeking nursing home work, long-term care facilities can better retain their staff. Later on in this report, we'll show you how to make this information work for you.

MYTH NUMBER 4:

Stress and burnout are no worse for nursing assistants than for any other worker.

If nursing assistants choose the job for all the right reasons, what happens? From our focus groups and surveys, we think we know the answer. Nursing assistants begin with a sense of enthusiasm, sound motivation, a desire to help others, and an interest in what appears to them to be a more "professional" job than might otherwise be available to them.

But, one might say, "a funny thing happens on the way to the bedpan...." Over time, otherwise motivated and energetic nursing assistants become burned out, and eventually leave.

How stressful is it to be a nursing assistant? Well, we have asked them. From our surveys, when asked "How stressful would you say your job is," only 10% say "not too stressful." Fourteen percent say it is "a little stressful." Fully 42% report that the work is "moderately stressful," and 34% say that it is "very stressful." That's a lot of people experiencing a lot of stress.

We have also administered a burnout inventory, scientifically developed for human service workers. The findings show that at least a third of the nursing assistants experience a seriously high rate of burnout.

Looking at some of the individual items in this scale that measures burnout, we can see how pervasive it is:

- 70% of nursing assistants say they feel burned out at least some of the time.

- 60% feel that they sometimes treat residents more impersonally than they would like.

- 40% feel that they have been hardened emotionally by the job.

Besides the obvious discomfort it causes for individual nursing assistants, it also causes problems for the facility as a whole. Why? **Because the greater the stress and burnout, the more likely your nursing assistants are to leave.** They may go to another nursing home where they think the pressure will be less, or they may leave nursing home work.

Some data from our surveys of nursing assistants make this point clearly. In addition to measuring stress and burnout, we also asked the nursing assistants how likely they were to quit their jobs soon. People who said they felt very burned out were more than twice as likely to say they were thinking of quitting in the near future. In fact, fully **56%** of the nursing assistants who said they were going to leave the facility soon were in the high burnout group.

The Four Major Causes of Stress and Burnout

Research has shown a number of causes of stress and burnout. Quite a bit has been written about this topic, and there are certainly a number of reasons. From our perspective, four major ones are as follows. In each case, the cause of stress is the **lack** of something important nursing assistants need.

1. Lack of Time

In our surveys, a third or more of the nursing assistants say that they routinely do not have enough time to complete their basic tasks. This sense of time pressure takes the enjoyment out of their work. Nursing assistants say that when time is short, they are not able to do the more personal, satisfying tasks, like walking with residents, talking to them, helping with personal care tasks, and so forth. When they feel like their job is reduced to the hardest, least gratifying tasks, and that they are always behind, they are much more likely to find their own solution — by **leaving.**

2. Lack of Staff

In the range of things that make staff dissatisfied, "working short" is among the most serious. It is clear that the staff who stay are often motivated by the affection they feel for their residents, and by the desire to be of service. The pressure caused by staff shortages is very severe, and makes nursing assistants feel like they can't do their jobs. In one study, adequate staffing was found to be the major factor that led to high staff morale.

Researcher Mary Ann Wilner has conducted extensive group discussions with nursing assistants. She found that a major source of dissatisfaction and stress was working with too few other nursing assistants, or with new staff who were not adequately trained. Nursing assistants were especially anxious about injury to themselves, to the rookie staff member, and to the residents in these situations.

Often, the most committed nursing assistants are the most disturbed by working short. They feel that they have to care for more residents in the same amount of time, and that the quality of care therefore suffers. Perhaps the most poignant comment came from one of Wilner's respondents. Because of a staff shortage, one of this nursing assistant's residents told her, "You don't like me any more!" because she had so little time to give the resident attention.

So "working short" is a major factor in nursing assistant stress. It can lead to poorer job performance, injuries, and staff burnout. It also drives staff to leave.

The problem of "working short" is one that we hope this report will help you with. By investigating your current situation and taking steps to improve, you will be able to retain staff longer, and slow down the revolving door.

3. Lack of Good Supervision

Nursing assistants often report that problems with supervisors are a major cause of burnout. As Mary Ann Wilner puts it, "Problems communicating with supervisors are often stressful. Nursing assistants feel like their opinions are sometimes not asked for, or that supervisors may talk down to them." Conflicts with supervisors are very upsetting to nursing assistants, especially when they feel powerless to change the situation.

How frequent are problems with supervisors? Theodore Helmer and his colleagues (1993) shed light on this question. They asked nursing assistants how they felt about the supervision they received and found the following:

- 71% wished administrators and nurses would show them more respect.

- Only 37% felt they received sufficient recognition and appreciation for their work.

- Only 36% felt that management makes them feel "in on things."

Supervision problems plague nursing homes, and help create nursing assistant turnover.

4. Lack of Preparation

We noted above that being a nursing assistant is not unskilled labor. It is a complicated job, that calls for the ability to negotiate many complicated situations. But the training given to nursing assistants is almost exclusively about the **technical** side of the job. It is the difficulty in dealing with the **psychosocial** aspects of nursing home work that causes stress, burnout, and leads to turnover.

I'll give you two examples here. These two characteristics of nursing home work have been found by researchers to be extremely stressful for nursing assistants. Then I want to give you a little test.

The first example is **death.** Unfortunately, a big part of a nursing assistant's job is dealing with death and dying. Favorite residents die, but the pressure of the work is too great to allow nursing assistants to grieve.

As death education expert Franne Whitney Nelson puts it, "Some residents may become as well loved by the nursing assistant as the nursing assistant's own family members. Nursing assistants can expect to feel grief, but most nursing homes don't create an environment in which nursing assistants can express their grief. The lack of opportunity for nursing assistants to mourn the death of a resident is one of the factors that contributes to the high rate of turnover among nursing assistants."

The second example is **aggression.** One of the most surprising findings of our surveys is the amount of conflict and aggression nursing assistants experience with residents. In our surveys, for example, 92% of nursing assistants report that they were pushed, grabbed, or shoved by a resident during the past year, and half of nursing assistants had this happen more than 10 times in the past year! About 70% had been hit or had something thrown at them, and fully 40% had been kicked or bitten.

Okay, here is the test: Did your facility have a good, serious, inservice training session on either of these topics in the past year? Not just a mention, but enough training so that your nursing assistants would really be better able to handle death and dying issues, or aggression from residents? Take a minute to think....

If you said yes to either one, you can pat yourself on the back (if you said yes to both, use both hands!) because you are in a tiny minority. These emotionally-laden problems are the kinds of issues that make or break a nursing assistant, not bathing techniques or infection control. And there are lots of other issues like this: dealing with family members, moral decisions, communication problems, and on and on.

Take a look at the box below. Cut it out. Hang it on your wall. And start thinking about what you're going to **do** about it.

LACK OF TIME + LACK OF STAFF + LACK OF GOOD SUPERVISION + LACK OF PREPARATION = STRESS AND BURNOUT = TURNOVER

MYTH NUMBER 5:

Nursing assistants are all the same.

There is a definite tendency to think that nursing assistants are all alike. We talk about "nursing assistants need..." or "nursing assistants want...." But we must realize that the nursing assistants have different backgrounds and characteristics.

William Crown and colleagues recently put together a national profile of nursing assistants. He found quite a bit of diversity.

- Despite the heavy concentration of younger nursing assistants — half are under the age of 35 — there is a fairly wide range of ages, with 10% age 55 or over.

- There is a much heavier concentration of minority workers in this occupation than in the rest of the workforce. About 30% of nursing assistants are members of minority groups.

- Although they are on average young, they are likely to have family responsibilities. Half are currently married, and another quarter are widowed, divorced, or separated. About half have at least one child under 18.

- Interestingly, the nursing home workforce is much better educated than we often assume. The majority (76%) have at least a high school education, and 16% have some kind of education beyond high school.

The moral here is: to solve recruitment and retention problems, one strategy may not be enough. We need to recognize that the work force is diverse, and explore multiple ways to attract and keep staff.

MYTH NUMBER 6:

Residents are concerned about the health care they receive, the surroundings, the food — not about the nursing assistants.

Everyone knows that nursing assistants provide most of the hands-on care in the nursing home. But their role is even more pivotal than that, however. As Genevieve Gipson puts it, "The nursing assistant is the point where the system touches the resident." It is this relationship that in large part determines the residents' experience.

But this is very easy to forget. Many people in the nursing home industry focus too heavily on the **technical** aspects of care when we think about quality. But, to put it bluntly, what residents primarily care about is not whether the light in the walk-in refrigerator is burned out, or precisely what the staff-to-resident ratio is, or how well you do your paperwork. Of course, those kinds of things are important, but most critical is what has been called the **interpersonal process.** How do living, breathing, human beings conduct relationships in the nursing home? How do people treat one another? This is what really counts.

Indeed, studies have shown that probably the most important thing in residents' overall well-being in the home is their relationships with staff. These day-to-day interactions with staff completely set the tone for their experience of life in the facility. Residents place greatest emphasis on these interpersonal aspects of care and on the amenities of care. Even if the technical aspects of care in a nursing home are carried out correctly, residents' experience of life in a nursing home may be negative. Long-term care residents view the facility as their home, where interpersonal interactions — especially those that occur with staff — become paramount. This, to residents, is the heart of quality care.

Compelling evidence for this point comes from a study done by the National Citizens' Coalition for Nursing Home Reform. They held small group discussions with 457 residents in 105 nursing homes throughout the country. In these discussions, relations with staff ranked far and away the most cited aspect of quality care. People noted that it was most important to have staff with good attitudes, who cared about them, and who treated them well.

More than improvements in environment, food service, or activities, residents valued staff who were kind, nice, and "good to them." They wanted staff to treat them with dignity, to be polite, to be friendly, cheerful, and pleasant. These kinds of factors, by the way, ranked far higher than being "qualified," or "skilled and knowledgeable."

So all of us must ask ourselves: do we focus enough on the interpersonal aspects of care? Do we allow relationships to develop between staff and residents? Do we have policies that disrupt relationships? And do we provide staff with the kind of training that will help them to have good relationships with residents? Because if we don't do these kinds of things, we are missing the major determinant of quality care, from the residents' perspective. And unless we do these things, we will not solve the turnover problem.

The Nursing Home Staffing "Golden Rule"

So these are the myths. What do they all add up to? We suggest that the way to combat these myths is something we call the nursing home staffing "Golden Rule."

This insight is something we have learned from nursing assistant expert Genevieve Gipson. She has found that people who stay in the job, who become "career" nursing assistants, are primarily motivated by the residents. Another way to put this is in psychological terms: The residents are the primary reinforcers for "career" nursing assistants. The satisfaction they receive from providing good care is what reinforces them. It is what makes them enjoy the job and find it worthwhile and meaningful.

When motivated, caring nursing assistants leave, it is not usually because of the wages or benefits. **Instead, they leave when they feel they can no longer do a good job.** If they do not have the time, the training, the supervision, or the physical supplies to properly care for their residents, they will eventually leave.

And so here is the "Golden Rule" that we will emphasize throughout the rest of this report:

Create an environment where
nursing assistants feel that
they can give good care.

The nursing assistants you want to attract and keep are motivated by the residents, and by what they can do to help them. What is really enjoyable for a nursing assistant is to offer kind, humane care, and to feel as if he or she is making a contribution to the resident's well-being. If you provide opportunities for these kinds of feelings, if you create an environment where the nursing assistant can give good care, your recruitment and retention problems will begin to disappear.

To help you create such an environment, we will next review the problem of turnover, and how you can get a handle on it in your facility.

CHAPTER FOUR

The Revolving Door
(and Why It Turns)

It is worth taking a moment to step back and think about your own (and your facility's) attitude toward nursing assistant turnover. How important do you consider turnover to be? In our discussions with administrators, we have seen a few common attitudes.

Some folks are genuinely concerned about the problem, and are trying to deal with it. But the most common attitude we have seen is what we would call "benign neglect." Administrators who fit into this mold see high rates of turnover in their facilities, but don't feel obliged to do anything about it, because enough new applicants seem to keep showing up at the door. Their attitude goes something like this: "Sure, it would be better not to have so much turnover, but it's not really hurting my operation."

So we first need to address the question: Is turnover bad?

This may seem like it has an obvious answer, but we should ask it anyway. After all, in some professions, turnover is considered positive — for example, in high-tech firms, computer specialists are expected to shift from one company to another. In universities, a common complaint is that, because of the tenure system, departments are full of "dead wood."

How Turnover Hurts

In nursing homes there is ample evidence that staff turnover has very negative consequences. If your turnover rate is high, your facility will be hit hard in three basic ways.

1. Financial

It is hard to put an exact dollar amount on the impact of turnover in nursing homes, because any estimate would vary by region, and salaries change so quickly that figures would become outdated. However, some experts suggest a rule of thumb for estimating turnover costs. In many occupations, according to this formula, four times the monthly salary of an employee is the likely cost. Using this formula as a guideline, the minimal replacement cost for a nursing assistant earning $6.00 per hour would be estimated at about $4,000.

Even if the costs are a little lower in your region, turnover is definitely expensive. Think about it: To replace a nursing assistant, you have to pay for all of the following:

- Advertising

- Checking references and background

- Setting up records for the new employee

- Orientation

- Training

- Lower productivity while the new hire learns the job

- Lower productivity of other staff, while they provide on-the-job training to the new hire.

You can probably add to this list.

2. Staff Morale

Researchers on turnover have found that a major source of satisfaction for employees is a sense of **integration.** That is, people get a sense of belonging from their work, if there is a stable group of work friends whom they know and trust. They feel like a part of a team in such a situation, and that is very satisfying for them.

For this reason, turnover rates lead to a vicious circle: The more staff who leave, the less contented are those staff persons who stay. Then these staff themselves become likely to leave. And of course, as we said earlier, chronic staff shortages lead to increased work load for nursing assistants, and more job stress.

In short, nothing is worse for staff morale than watching the revolving door spin.

3. Quality of Care

Probably the residents suffer the most from high turnover rates. Study after study has demonstrated the critical importance of continuity of care for residents. Their lives are often characterized by a sense of lack of control, and by anxiety over the frightening changes that are going on in their own bodies. These feelings in turn lead residents to want a stable and predictable environment.

For this reason, the revolving door has a very detrimental impact on the quality of resident care. The researcher Barbara Bowers has amply demonstrated that new staff do not provide as competent care; when there is a continual stream of new staff, care certainly will suffer.

Jean Kruzich and her colleagues found strong evidence for this assertion in an interesting piece of research. In a survey of 289 residents in 51 nursing homes, they found that there was a direct relationship between resident satisfaction with the facility and the average length of employment of the nursing assistants. That is, the longer nursing assistants stayed on the job, the more satisfied the residents were. (This also applied to nursing staff, by the way; the higher the RN turnover rate, the lower the residents' satisfaction.)

To put it simply, in the nursing home setting there is nothing good to be said about a high turnover rate. Turnover is like taxes: the lower, the better. To begin to reduce turnover, your first weapon is knowledge. To understand your facility's turnover problem, you have to answer two key questions: **How much?** and **Why?**

Measuring Turnover in Your Facility

My main goal in this chapter is to convince you of one fact: What you don't know **will** hurt you! In our conversations throughout the country, we have been amazed by how few facilities track their turnover rates.

What about you? Take the following little quiz:

1. The turnover rate for nursing assistants in my facility last quarter was _____.

2. The turnover rate for nursing assistants in my facility for the past year was _____.

3. Over the past three years, the turnover rate in my facility has:

    a) gone up

    b) gone down

    c) stayed the same.

If you were able to answer these questions off the top of your head, congratulate yourself: Many facilities have no idea about this critically important statistic.

One of the strongest recommendations in this report is that **every facility should calculate its CNA turnover rate every quarter.** Closely monitoring your turnover rate can help you get a handle on problems in your facility, and can also help you to estimate staffing needs. When you combine this statistical information with exit interviews with staff who leave (see below), you can get a very good picture of your turnover situation.

Calculating Turnover Rates

Marguerite Birkenstock has laid out how to calculate turnover in a very clear way; we have adapted her method more specifically for nursing assistants. First we present the basic steps, and then we work out an example for you.

> **STEP 1.** Using your employee records, determine the average number of nursing assistants who were on the payroll for the past quarter. To get this number, take the number of nursing assistants who were on the payroll on the last day of each month in the quarter, then divide by the number of months (for a quarter, this would be three months).

> **STEP 2.** Determine from your employee records how many nursing assistants left your facility during the quarter.

STEP 3. Take the number of nursing assistants who left during the quarter, and divide it by the average number of nursing assistants on the payroll during the same quarter. Then you multiply it by 100 to get the turnover rate. For those of you who like formulas, it looks like this:

$$\frac{\text{NUMBER OF CNAs WHO LEFT DURING THE QUARTER}}{\text{AVERAGE NUMBER OF CNAs ON PAYROLL FOR QUARTER}} \times 100 = \text{TURNOVER RATE}$$

Armed with this quarterly data, you can track nursing assistant turnover rates over time. You can also add up the quarterly rates and calculate an annual rate.

EXAMPLE: GOODCARE NURSING HOME

It's April, and the administrator at Goodcare Nursing Home is fighting spring fever. She decides that now is a good time to start tracking turnover in her facility. She collects her management team around the table, and armed with staffing records, they proceed to calculate CNA turnover for the first quarter of the year (January, February, and March). Here's what happens:

STEP 1: Calculate Average Number of Nursing Assistants on Payroll for the Quarter.

Looking at the employee records, they find out the number of nursing assistants who were employed on the last day of each of the three months. It looks like this:

January 31	=	50
February 29	=	45
March 31	=	55
TOTAL	**=**	**150**

Next, they divide this number (150) by the number of months (3). So they come up with an average number of nursing assistants on the payroll during the quarter of 50.

STEP 2: Determine How Many Nursing Assistants Left During the Quarter.

This is determined from the paperwork on exiting staff. It turns out that five nursing assistants left the facility during the quarter.

STEP 3: Calculate the Turnover Rate.

This is easily done, using the formula we showed above, since we have all the data:

$$\frac{5}{50} = .10 \times 100 = 10\%$$

And there you have it: your quarterly turnover rate for the first three months is 10%.

Now, let's say the staff at Goodcare does their job, and keeps on calculating the quarterly rates for the whole year. They come up with the following data:

First quarter   = 10%

Second quarter = 7%

Third quarter   = 5%

Fourth quarter = 3%

Add those four numbers up, and you get the annual turnover rate at Goodcare: 25%.

The Next Step: Who is Turning Over?

Once you have these basic numbers, you can refine them to learn more about turnover. For example, you may want to look at turnover rates for different types of employees. It is particularly useful to look at **who** is turning over.

For example, it may be that much of the turnover is occurring among new nursing assistants. This stands to reason, since it is during the early months that nursing assistants are finding out whether they like the work. But if there is high turnover of new staff, you may need to look especially carefully at your training and orientation program (see Chapter 5).

You would have a different problem if it is your longer-term, more experienced staff who are leaving. This could point to dissatisfaction with changes in your facility, or competition from other employers. Responses here might include wage improvements, job redesign, or career ladders (see Chapter 7).

As this example shows, when it comes to turnover, knowledge is power. The more you know about nursing assistant turnover in your facility, the better you can target your efforts to fight it.

Exit Interviews

But this only begins to answer the question: **Why** do nursing assistants leave? Fortunately, there is a simple answer to this question: **Ask them!** One of the major surprises for us as we have traveled around the country talking with administrators is how frequently they fail to take this step. Your staff are the best sources of information about why turnover occurs in your facility — but only if you ask them.

The best way to investigate the causes of turnover is the **exit interview.** You can be greatly helped by surveying and interviewing nursing assistants who leave. We tend to equate turnover with job dissatisfaction, and that is not necessarily true. Take, for example, a community that is almost completely dominated by a large university. Many graduate students and postdoctoral researchers come there for one or two years. Their spouses look for work, stay a year or two, and then leave. If you looked at the turnover rates at many employers in that city, they would likely be quite high, but that may well have nothing to do with dissatisfaction.

In a nursing home, people leave for all kinds of reasons: job dissatisfaction, a spouse gets a new job, they have a baby, they move too far way, and so on. If you've got a problem with turnover, you need to find out why. And this is where the exit interview comes in.

The management consultant Bill Marvin has done excellent work in this area, and several of his ideas are worth noting.

Exit interviewing is an inexpensive way to get a sense of what's going on in your organization, and it's also a very effective way. In general, a departing employee has nothing to lose by being honest, and therefore is a great source of information.

However, on the flip side, there may be some exiting employees who are leaving because they are angry at management, or who are worried that they may need a recommendation from the facility, and so won't be open about their feelings to someone in the nursing home.

Marvin suggests getting someone from outside the facility who will be seen as "safe" to talk to. In large multifacility operations, the personnel office may be able to fulfill that function. But for many other facilities, it can work well to hire a person as needed to interview departing employees. A good choice might be an experienced nurse or nursing assistant who has retired or left to raise a family, but would like some part-time work.

An interview with such a person can be an excellent source of information, because the interviewer can make the person feel comfortable and draw out the reasons why they are leaving. The major difficulty lies in coordinating schedules so that the exit interview can take place. It may help to pay the departing employee $5 or $10 for completing the interview. An alternative is using a survey form for departing employees. The key thing is to get the information in some way. Here are some sample questions you can use to survey departing nursing assistants:

SAMPLE EXIT INTERVIEW QUESTIONS

1. Why did you decide to leave at this time?

2. How important were these factors in making you decide to stop working in this facility? Circle the number below the answer.

		VERY IMPORTANT	SOMEWHAT IMPORTANT	NOT IMPORTANT
A.	Commuting time	3	2	1
B.	Change in family responsibilities (e.g., new child)	3	2	1
C.	Dissatisfied with the wages here	3	2	1
D.	Problems with my supervisor/s	3	2	1
E.	Too much job stress	3	2	1
F.	Dissatisfied with the benefits here	3	2	1
G.	Problems with my co-workers	3	2	1
H.	Tired of nursing home work	3	2	1
I.	Poor opportunities for advancement	3	2	1
J.	Other _____			

3. Is there anything that would have made you decide to continue to work here longer? If so, what is it?

4. If you could change anything you wanted to in this facility, what would it be?

5. Would you recommend this facility to someone who was interested in becoming a nursing assistant? Why or why not?

You also do not need to limit your efforts to departing staff. We highly recommend conducting occasional surveys of your current employees. You can easily develop a set of questions that can be given to nursing assistants. Even a few questions that you and other administrative staff can review will be very helpful. Focus group discussions can also be very useful, especially when you can get a neutral person from outside the facility conduct them.

The moral here is: Get the information you need to understand what is causing your recruitment and retention problems. Talk to the staff, and learn from them — even if the answers are a little painful at the start!

Now that you understand why your staff leave, you are ready to address the next challenge — finding the talented and dedicated staff you need.

CHAPTER FIVE

Recruiting for Excellence

To reduce turnover and create a committed, stable nursing assistant workforce, let's take our motto from Ben Franklin's *Poor Richard's Almanac:* "An ounce of prevention is worth a pound of cure." In the long run, it will cost you a whole lot less to attract the right kind of people than it does to keep on hiring new ones. The goal is to get the best person for the job; do this, and some of your employee retention problems will disappear. To borrow from the military, your goal should be to look for "a few good women and men."

To recruit excellent nursing assistants, there are three basic steps:

1. **Get the word out:** Creatively build public awareness about the benefits of working in your facility.

2. **Choose carefully:** A rigorous staff selection process will help ensure that you have the best nursing assistants.

3. **Start new staff on the right foot:** Orientation is key to successfully completing the recruitment process.

As you can see, these steps imply an approach to recruitment that goes far beyond putting an ad in the newspaper and waiting for the phone to ring. Our research makes it clear that recruitment doesn't stop when the applicant enters the door. Simply filling a slot is not going to solve your problem over the long term. If a person leaves after one, or three, or six months, this may be the worst scenario: the time and resources invested in training are wasted.

So let's explore some possible solutions to recruitment problems. Some of these ideas are quite simple, while others are more complex and require the cooperation of other facilities or organizations. All are well worth a try.

Step 1: Get the Word Out

To get good nursing assistants, you have to ask people. This point may seem obvious, but let's take a lesson from a story told about the late Speaker of the House, Tip O'Neill.

In one of his first runs for office in Massachusetts, Tip lost by only a few votes. Shortly thereafter, he was talking to a lifelong neighbor about the election. This was a woman whose walk he had shoveled and whose groceries he had delivered; a sure vote, he thought. But she admitted she hadn't voted for him. Tip was dumbfounded. He nearly shouted: "But Mrs. O'Grady — after everything I've done for you, how could you not have voted for me?" To which she responded: "Well, Tip, you never asked me!"

Ask yourself and your staff the same question. Do we do a good job of asking people in the community if they are interested in working as a nursing assistant? Does the community know about our facility? Are they aware of what work is like in the facility? What do we do beyond placing a "help wanted" ad in the newspaper? Creatively brainstorm about this issue, and you will probably come up with a number of ideas about how better to get the word out.

Five Easy Suggestions

To get you started, here are five suggestions that facilities have had success with.

1. **Recruit at local job fairs.**
   Many communities have such events, and an attractive exhibit at a job fair can help bring in new recruits. High schools and vocational schools often sponsor such events. Community health fairs are also a good place to recruit. Consider sponsoring a job fair with other health care providers in your community or region.

2. **Hold open houses in your facility.**
   It is amazing how many neighborhood residents walk by a nursing home, wonder about it for a moment, and then walk on. Some of those individuals might be very interested in nursing home work: women re-entering the labor force, displaced homemakers, and parents looking for part-time jobs are only a few of the possibilities. Even if attendance is small at an open house, the word will spread surprisingly quickly.

3. **Use the media.**

   Get yourself in the paper, or on the radio (or even on TV!). Issue a press release to the local media about the shortage of nursing assistants in your community. Arrange for coverage of special events in your facility, such as Career Nurse Assistants Day (see below). For help in approaching the media, take a look at any of the popular books on marketing available in your local library or bookstore (*Guerrilla Marketing Attack,* by Jay Levinson, has especially good information on getting into the media). Because that is what you are doing: using the media to market to potential employees.

4. **Use your current nursing assistants to help you recruit new ones.**

   A number of facilities have successfully offered bonuses to staff if they recruit someone who is eventually hired. Such recruits are more likely to stay on the job, as well, because they have a supportive friend in the facility who can help them.

5. **Enlist the help of family members.**

   Let the family members of your residents know that there are opportunities for nursing assistants. They know your facility well, and can help you spread the word about job openings.

The moral here is: Don't be afraid to start out small. Activities like these can have a snowball effect, leading to an increased number of applicants.

Thinking Bigger

Beyond these smaller steps, a very effective approach is to conduct a large-scale public awareness campaign. Such an effort is based on the fact that the general public does not have a good understanding of what working in a nursing home is like (even worse, people often have a negative impression). Some state associations have combated this problem by conducting media campaigns to interest people in becoming nursing assistants.

The Massachusetts Extended Care Federation successfully used just such an approach. A few years ago, they started the first statewide campaign in the country to promote nursing home employment. This campaign also sought to improve the overall image and status of nursing home employees.

The campaign used a combination of broadcast and print advertising, urging people, in the campaign's slogan, to "make more than a living, make a difference." The television spots featured employees from Massachusetts nursing homes talking about their own work experiences.

According to the Massachusetts Federation, the campaign was successful in a number of ways. Their research showed that public awareness of the campaign was high. Hundreds of calls from potential employees were made to an 800 number set up for the campaign. An interesting side effect of the effort, beyond generating new applicants, was the impact on current staff. Many nursing home workers who saw the spots felt that they enhanced their self-esteem, and made them feel good about their work. (So don't forget: a recruitment strategy can have an impact on retention, as well!)

I know that such a project may seem far out of your reach at the moment. But remember: Desperate times call for desperate measures! As we said earlier, lots of other employers — home health agencies, day care centers, restaurants, hotels, and more — are competing for the same employees you are. Now may be the time for you to invest some time and energy, perhaps with other facilities or your state association, to plan a larger-scale recruitment campaign.

However you approach it, keep this in mind: The more people who know about the possible rewards of work as a nursing assistant, the more job applicants you will have.

Help Create a New Workforce

One more way to ensure a supply of new, qualified nursing assistants is also a "big ticket" item. That is, it takes time and energy on your part, and some creative thinking. But in my opinion, any facility (or group of cooperating facilities) that takes this approach will benefit for years to come. By working with community educational institutions, you can generate a continual supply of trained nursing assistants.

The key here is **to look in the right place for employees.** Remember the point I made earlier: Nursing assistant work can provide excellent opportunities for certain groups of people. However, we need to work with these population groups to interest them in nursing home work, and to train them so they succeed in it. In communities around the country, training partnerships have been developed that are helping to relieve the scarcity of nursing assistants.

Here are just three examples that have worked:

1. Students
A vocational high school trains students for elder care careers. Students are offered an elective course in their senior year. They receive 60 hours of classroom instruction and 15 hours of practicum. They then take the certification exam.

2. Older Adults
An excellent program trains older adults for work in long-term care. This makes sense: Many persons over the age of 55 are looking for work, sometimes after retirement, or, for women, after widowhood or divorce (so-called "displaced homemakers"). This approach has one clear advantage: Research shows that older nursing assistants are more likely to be reliable, to have higher job satisfaction, and are less likely to leave the job after a short time. In collaboration with nursing homes, a university developed a 200 hour curriculum, with field experience, for older persons.

3. Displaced Workers

Persons who are unemployed or on welfare can also be targeted. Such programs will have great potential during the coming years, as public policy tries to move people out of the welfare system. Model programs screen participants, and counsel them throughout the training period. Classroom training is mixed with on-the-job experience, guided by a "peer mentor."

Of course, it can be time-consuming to start programs such as these. But inquiries to a local university or high school may get someone interested in taking on the lion's share of the effort. One advantage to such programs is that federal, state, and private foundation funds may be available to cover all or part of the costs.

So, what does "getting the word out" mean? Basically, it means that we have to stop focusing only on the short term — how will I have enough nursing assistants next week? — and begin to focus on long-term solutions — how can I develop an excellent pool of nursing assistants over the next few years?

Step 2: Choose Carefully

What does your facility do to screen potential employees? Do you go beyond a cursory background and references check to find out if the applicant will really make a good, long-term, nursing assistant? If we fail to carry out a more thorough screening, we shouldn't be surprised when we wind up with inappropriate or uncommitted employees.

As a beginning step, try to expand your initial interview with applicants. It is surprising how many facilities do not ask basic questions about care-giving experience. Studies have found that people who have had some kind of experience caring for a dependent person are more likely to be satisfied as a nursing assistant, whether it is in a paid position, or as an informal caregiver for an elderly relative, a younger sibling, or someone else.

Other questions should be included that examine the fit between the applicant and the job. For example, someone who requires a rigid routine on the job may not be ideally suited to be a nursing assistant, because crises often unpredictably disrupt the work day. Similarly, someone who is uncomfortable with death and dying issues is unlikely to become a long-term employee.

In addition, consider adding a tour of the facility to the interview experience. If possible, let the applicant see nursing assistants at work (or better yet, talk with them) before he or she makes a decision. Some people have an idealized vision of "helping the elderly," which does not match up entirely with the day-to-day reality of the job.

"Nursing Assistant Test Battery"

An excellent example of a nursing assistant screening system comes from the Franciscan Health Care System in Dayton, Ohio. Plagued by high turnover rates at their facilities, Franciscan decided to experiment with more extensive staff screening. They had the logical idea that if they could select nursing assistants who were committed to a long-term relationship with the organization, and who had the potential for excellence in a demanding job, they would have an improved workforce.

To accomplish this goal, they developed a questionnaire called the "Nursing Assistant Test Battery." This interview taps five important dimensions:

1. Cognitive skills (such as understanding directions)

2. Administrative skills (such as being able to organize)

3. Interpersonal skills (such as likability and cooperation, compassion, and consideration)

4. Motivation (such as personal pride and enthusiasm)

5. Adjustment (such as reliability and responsibility).

According to Franciscan, this detailed screening procedure worked wonders. Their turnover rate dropped, and nursing assistant performance improved. Even if you are not ready to introduce such a formal screening method, try expanding your applicant interviews to help you select the best people.

Step 3: Start New Staff on the Right Foot

Before we move on to some suggestions to improve retention of employees, there is one more important point about the recruitment process. Let's say that you have been successful at recruiting and screening some interested new nursing assistants, and you have a full classroom on the first day of training. The recruitment process is still not over!

A crucial fact is this: **When you begin staff training, you are still recruiting.** That is, the first impressions the new staff have about the facility and the job are absolutely critical. Some facilities have reported that as many as 80% of new hires leave during the orientation period.

Harry Everett makes an excellent suggestion: Place a major emphasis on "starting out on the right foot." This means, he proposes, that we should pay special attention to a new hire's first day. This sets the tone for the future, and affects whether the new person will stay on. The goal is to show the new staff person how much he or she is individually valued by the facility.

Day One

Some effective strategies on the first day at the facility, according to Everett, include:

- Give each new employee a clear and detailed orientation package, including a schedule for the first day on the job, information about the goals of the orientation, a timetable for the first shift, and a good description of the actual work that will be done with residents.

- Have the administrator personally introduce each new nursing assistant during a meal on the first shift, and say a few words about how important the new person is.

- Make it clear to each new hire where he or she can get help. Clearly identify a staff person to whom the new person can go with questions or to ask for help. Develop a "buddy system," where an experienced nursing assistant is paired with a new hire for support and advice.

- Don't devote all of the first day to classroom training. Make sure that the new nursing assistant has a chance to perform a few of the job's basic tasks on the first day.

To sum up: Be creative and imaginative in your efforts to attract frontline staff. See the training period as continuing recruitment. Using these ideas will help you end the recruitment process with committed new nursing assistants.

Your next task will be to nurture and sustain that commitment. Let's look at some ways to do that.

CHAPTER SIX

Recognizing Real Worth

To say that nursing assistants feel unrecognized and underappreciated is probably the understatement of the year. In our focus groups and surveys, we have heard statements like this hundreds of times: "We always hear right away when we have done something wrong. But we never hear about it when we do something right!"

Decades of studies about how people learn, and how they change their behavior, should have taught us by now one simple truth: People can be motivated to improve their performance much more effectively through rewards than through punishment and criticism.

It's really quite simple: If you consistently recognize good performance among your staff, you will keep them much longer. Therefore, you need to ask yourself, and your supervisory staff, the following question: How do we recognize good performance by nursing assistants in my facility?

Informal Recognition

First, think about how you recognize employees **informally.** Supervisory staff should be sure to congratulate nursing assistants for good care on a regular basis. Make this a rule in your facility:

> *Every supervisory staff member must*
> *point out and publicly praise at least one*
> *action by a nursing assistant every day.*

Don't just stop there. When someone does something well, put it in writing! Administrators and directors of nursing should send a nursing assistant a note or letter if he or she performs in an outstanding way. A good occasion for such a note is when a family member reports a positive thing a nursing assistant has done.

In a word: praise, praise, praise. And do it **in public** whenever you can.

Formal Recognition

Equally important is a **formal** recognition system. Here are several possibilities for structured recognition programs in a nursing home.

Supervisor Evaluation

An incentive system can be based on supervisor ratings of nursing assistant performance. Charge nurses, for example, can evaluate nursing assistants in a variety of areas, including personal care skills, respect for residents, and interaction with families. Nursing assistants who meet a previously established standard are then rewarded with recognition within the facility (such as having their name on a plaque, or their photograph displayed), and with a gift, such as voucher for a dinner in a restaurant, a gift certificate to a local store, or something similar.

Peer Evaluation

In this type of program, staff are recognized based on an evaluation by their peers. This has the advantage of empowering the nursing assistants themselves to recognize one another. An example of such a program is the Episcopal Church Home of Minnesota's "Caught in the Act of Caring" program. Nominations come from other workers, and the person with the most nominations each month receives a gift certificate to a local store or restaurant.

Facility-wide Recognition

In addition to recognizing individual employees, a wonderful idea is to devote one day during the year to "celebrating the nursing assistant." The most complete recognition program of this type has been developed by Genevieve Gipson, who has spent over two decades seeking to improve the work life of nursing assistants. She is now the director of the Career Nurse Assistants Program, which promotes opportunities to recognize nursing assistants.

Career Nurse Assistants Day

The most visible part of this effort is Career Nurse Assistants Day. In the words of Gipson, it "is a special day set aside each year to celebrate the experience of the career nurse assistant, by recognizing the role, accomplishments, and value of this important worker to the resident and the health care system." Each year, hundreds of nursing homes throughout the country take part in Career Nurse Assistants Day.

Many facilities obtain a proclamation from the mayor of their town or city. This then serves as a trigger for other activities. The facility can publicize the proclamation and issue news articles around the fact that the mayor has proclaimed the official day. Most facilities then have award ceremonies, essay contests, fashion shows, or other events.

The benefits of Career Nurse Assistants Day are many. The facility obtains considerable publicity, and can project a positive image in the community. Family members of residents, and the residents themselves, appreciate the events. And, of course, staff satisfaction increases.

Consistent and regular employee recognition is simply a part of good management in any organization. But it is especially important in the nursing home setting. Our research has shown that nursing assistants tend to feel **disempowered**. Although they do a demanding job, and often identify strongly with their work, they do not have many of the sources of recognition and self-esteem that professionals do. They do not subscribe to professional journals, attend management seminars, or go to conferences. On-the-job recognition can thus have especially powerful effects for nursing assistants.

Use Your Creativity

To administrators and supervisors, we would say: Have **fun** with recognition! Use your imagination and creativity. Brainstorm with the nursing assistants themselves about how **they** would like to be recognized.

To get you going, let's take a look at human resources expert Robert L. Desatnick's suggestions in his excellent book *Keep the Customer*. Here, I've adapted some of his ideas, drawn from Fortune 500 firms, to the nursing home.

EIGHT RECOGNITION IDEAS

1. **Internal contests,** where staff on different units compete to be the best in some area (e.g., low absenteeism) during a given time period.

2. **Employee of the month** and unit of the month recognition programs.

3. Solicit **letters of recognition** from family members and display them in the facility's entrance or lounge and send copies to local media, legislators, and Governor's and Mayor's offices.

4. **Publish stories** of outstanding service by nursing assistants in facility publications, such as newsletters.

5. Place a **special recognition symbol** on an employee's name badge for outstanding job performance

6. Sponsor **staff parties and trips** on a regular basis.

7. **Rookie of the month.** Every month (or quarter) recognize a new employee for outstanding service. Have an award ceremony attended by other nursing assistants.

8. And a last, fascinating idea: Nursing assistants vote for a **"Supervisor of the Year."** This allows them to identify and reward good job performance.

To sum up: Everyone says that nursing assistants are the "unsung heroes" of the long-term care world. But why should they be **unsung?** If you create a climate in your nursing home where excellence is consistently recognized, I can guarantee that the work atmosphere will improve. This, in turn, will lower turnover and increase job satisfaction among nursing assistants.

Let's turn our attention now to some successful strategies designed to recognize, encourage, and support staff.

CHAPTER SEVEN

Three "Best Practices" to Retain Nursing Assistants

One of my main goals in this report is to argue that the vicious cycle of nursing assistant turnover can be turned into a positive feed-back loop. Perhaps another way to think about turnover is to replace the image of a revolving door with that of an escalator. Instead of a cycle of staff shortages which leads to burnout which, in turn, leads to turnover, we can move to an upward progression, in which committed nursing assistants receive support, are allowed increased professionalism and mastery in their jobs, and can advance to positions of greater responsibility.

It is important to remember that recruitment and retention are not really two separate activities. Instead, they represent a seamless web of concern for the development of the nursing assistant. Everything you do to upgrade the working conditions of your nursing assistants will help you in recruitment. The word quickly spreads in a community, and more applicants will begin to show up if your facility gets the reputation as a place that "really cares" about nursing assistants.

For example, one nursing home we know had a very high turnover rate and a lot of trouble attracting applicants for nursing assistant jobs. Then a new director of nursing came on board, who decided to try some changes. She did some of the things we discuss in the following pages, like involving nursing assistants in decision-making and developing career ladder programs. Even though the facility did not raise salaries, the word quickly got around that this nursing home was a more congenial place to work, and the number of applicants picked up.

In this chapter, we focus on three "best practices" that we have identified in our exploration of programs around the nation. Each of these programs involves re-thinking the needs of nursing assistants and the nature of their job. In each case, the payoffs in decreased turnover and increased staff satisfaction are potentially very great.

BEST PRACTICE NUMBER 1:

Career Ladder Programs

Sometimes in the nursing home world, we do not need expensive studies with fancy statistics to tell us basic truths. Instead we only need common sense: one major cause of turnover is that we offer nursing assistants "no place to go — but out!"

Over and over, when you ask nursing assistants what they don't like about their jobs, you hear: "There's no place to go. It's a dead end." There is no doubt that if we want to retain good nursing assistants, there has to be some way for them to go up a ladder of increasing responsibility. Otherwise, they stagnate and eventually leave.

Think about your own career. How would you feel if there was no possibility for advancement, nothing to work toward? Would you stay in such a job for long? Unfortunately, we tend to act in a contradictory way: We want career nursing assistants, but we do not actually offer them a career.

To be sure, some facilities have scholarship programs to allow nursing assistants to pursue the goal of becoming a nurse. Project LINC in New York City is perhaps the most extensive program of this kind. It funds nursing assistants to attend nursing school, and provides them with support while they attend school. Such programs benefit not only the individual, but can also help us solve the long-term care nursing shortage.

However, these programs do not help us solve the **nursing assistant** shortage. Indeed, they move talented nursing assistants into supervisory positions. Further, many nursing assistants we have talked to do not wish to become nurses. They enjoy the contact they have with residents, and are not interested in what they see as a managerial position that involves much paperwork. They would like opportunities to advance, but still remain in the profession of nursing assistant.

One of the most exciting innovations in nursing home care is the design of nursing assistant "career ladder" programs. Such programs not only benefit the staff, who feel they can progress and grow, they also benefit the facility, by preparing nursing assistants to meet the increased demands of heavier care residents.

One Company's Approach

One of the most comprehensive programs of this kind was developed at Genesis Eldercare (formerly Genesis Health Ventures) in Pennsylvania. Carolyn McDonald, formerly of Genesis and now an educational consultant in Massachusetts, was integral to the development of the Genesis career ladder, and has described it in several articles.

McDonald emphasizes that the career ladder is very flexible, and that a nursing home can design it in many ways. In the Genesis program, the first rung of the ladder is called the Geriatric Nursing Assistant Specialist. To be eligible for the program, candidates must work in the facility for at least six months, and must have had an above average performance evaluation. A six-month training program is then provided through a local community college. The program is made up of six modules, for a total of 108 hours. Upon completion, there is a formal graduation.

Data collected in February, 1996 reveals that since 1988 when the GNAS program began, more than 1200 nursing assistants have completed it. The overall rate of retention is 72%.

Some nursing assistants decide to remain at this rung of the ladder, but there is a second step, as well. This is the Senior Nursing Assistant, who serves as a team leader for the nursing assistants on the unit. For this position, the nursing assistants take 30 hours of leadership training. They help solve problems at a more basic level than nurses are able to.

At the top of the ladder is the Senior Aide Coordinator. This person serves as a team leader and role model for all the nursing assistants in the facility. The Coordinator attends department meetings, helps with orientation, and serves as a liaison to families. He or she also meets with all nursing assistants in the facility regularly.

Genesis reported dramatic reductions in turnover and improved morale. They had more job applicants, because of the possibilities for advancement. It should be noted that modest salary increases accompany the completion of the course and advancement to each new position.

This model is tremendously exciting. It helps to solve many of the sources of dissatisfaction and turnover discussed earlier. It gives nursing assistants hope for the future and something to work toward, and helps to ensure a stable workforce. Even if such a structured program is not right for you at the moment, brainstorm with your staff to come up with at least one or two ways in which nursing assistants can be promoted.

Most important, such programs show the kind of respect for nursing assistants that is greatly needed. Human resources expert Robert Desatnick sums this point up beautifully: "The best reward for high achievement is to give the individual the opportunity to do more."

BEST PRACTICE NUMBER 2:

Increasing Peer Support

As we noted earlier in this report, research has demonstrated that the degree of satisfaction with co-worker relationships is a strong predictor of turnover in nursing homes. As research has shown, if staff do not feel integrated with and supported by co-workers, they are more likely to leave.

Indeed, our studies and those of others have shown that a major problem nursing assistants experience is a lack of support from their peers. All too often, they feel isolated in their work, unable to connect with others, or sometimes even in competition with other nursing assistants.

It is critical to establish a cooperative atmosphere among nursing assistants. One issue to be aware of is the rotation of staff. Research has shown that greater staff integration is one effect of permanent assignment of a group of staff to a particular unit or group of residents. The rotation model of staffing, where nursing assistants are regularly assigned to new units with new co-workers, can make nursing assistants feel more isolated. In permanent assignment models, staff not only develop closer relationships with residents, but also with other nursing assistants with whom they share a long-term relationship.

Of course, a shift to permanent assignment of staff may not be possible at this point in your facility. However, when making staff assignments, try to keep the following point in mind: Most people prefer continuity in their co-worker relationships. Having to develop new relationships to a new group three or four times a year adds to the stress of the nursing assistant's job.

A second point is one we have mentioned earlier: Establish "buddy systems" in your facility. Consider allowing nursing assistants to pair up on the job. This is especially critical in the early stages of a nursing assistant's career. Providing each new nursing assistant with a "peer mentor" can make the entry into nursing home work much easier. (And remember Chapter 6: Don't forget to formally recognize the "peer mentor" for taking on this responsibility!)

Support Groups

A more comprehensive way to address this issue is the nursing assistant support group program, developed by Mary Ann Wilner. In a research project she conducted, Wilner found that the intense job pressure often makes nursing assistants isolated. She noted that the isolation is increased by the lack of opportunities to exchange information with peers on the job.

Wilner's project placed experienced group leaders in 16 nursing homes. The evaluation showed that the groups helped the nursing assistants to work better as a team, to learn from each other, and to develop new coping skills. Many members reported an increase in self-confidence and reduced stress. Modest reductions in turnover were also found in the facilities that used the program.

Wilner suggests the following points to make a support group successful:

SUPPORT GROUP GUIDELINES

- Include only nursing assistants, to ensure a comfortable, uninhibited discussion.

- Membership must be voluntary; no one should be forced to attend the support group.

- Limit the group size to 15 members.

- Initially invite all nursing assistants, so everyone feels included. If more than 15 are interested, start another group.

- After the fourth meeting, close the membership, to allow group solidarity to develop.

- Keep all discussions totally confidential. Be sure to hold meetings in a private room.

- Topics for discussion are generated by the nursing assistants, not the administration. This is peer support, not a didactic training program.

- Use an experienced group leader from outside the facility. Avoid using the facility social worker or another employee, because confidentially must be assured. Places to find group leaders include schools of social work, local psychotherapists, and clinical social workers.

Like all retention programs, the support group concept requires full support from the administrator, director of nursing, and charge nurses. According to Wilner, "People have to have the attitude that even if there's an emergency, you don't cancel the support group." Making a consistent room available and providing refreshments also promotes the success of the group.

BEST PRACTICE NUMBER 3:

Job Redesign

In recent years, an increasing number of nursing homes have been taking a hard look at how the work of nursing assistants is organized. Some facilities have begun to experiment with different models of supervision for nursing assistants, in an effort to bring them into the decision-making process. Based on our review, such programs have major potential to reduce turnover.

Specifically, as was pointed out in Chapter 3, nursing assistants who stay in the job tend to be more satisfied with supervision, and, conversely, poor supervision is a big reason why nursing assistants become dissatisfied. Supervisors who are flexible and listen to nursing assistants are major sources of satisfaction.

Compelling evidence for the importance of supervision comes from Mary Ann Wilner's study. In her groups, problems communicating with supervisors was one of the most frequently discussed topics. Nursing assistants felt that when they raise problems to nurses, they are seen as gossiping or complaining, or even as being insubordinate. More often, supervisors simply do not ask nursing assistants' opinions. The nursing assistants felt that their knowledge of the residents was not being tapped, and that the residents were suffering as a result. A commonly offered example was the unhappiness that results for residents because the nursing assistants are not consulted about roommate assignments.

They also felt that residents suffer because vital information is not communicated to them from supervisors. They might not be informed, for example, about medical changes in residents who have recently returned from a hospital. Overall, anxiety about talking to nurses, and confusion about how to handle supervisors who treat them condescendingly, occupied much discussion time in the group.

One solution to these supervision problems is job redesign. Making the nursing assistants active participants in redesigning their work life can be a very effective tool to increase satisfaction with supervision, and with the work environment in general.

Unfortunately, there is still a lack of practical experience in the long-term care industry. Although a number of other industries have developed new ways of designing frontline jobs, so far only a few attempts have been made in nursing homes. But we do know enough to state definitively that participatory job redesign can help improve job satisfaction and reduce turnover.

What Is Job Redesign?

Diane Brannon provides a clear definition, suggesting that the term refers to "the deliberate restructuring of tasks and task sequences to provide more stimulating and motivating work, and to generate more productive use of staff resources." To this I would add, restructuring of tasks **with the input and influence of nursing assistants.**

The major suggestion of those who have worked on job redesign in long-term care is this: Nursing assistants should be made **active participants** in decisions about their work. A major source of dissatisfaction, as noted above, is the feeling on the part of many nursing assistants that they have no input into decision-making processes.

This situation is very unfortunate, because nursing assistants are an immensely valuable resource for continuous improvement of the quality of care in the facility. They have the most intimate knowledge of the residents, and wherever greater involvement has been tried, they have been able to solve care-related problems. In fact, one recent study found that nursing assistants who planned to stay on in the facility were much more likely to say that they were involved in care planning.

Incremental Approaches

The term "job redesign" may sound like it implies a major effort to transform your facility. Although some facilities have had great success with major changes (see below), small-scale attempts at empowering nursing assistants to find solutions to work problems are in fact highly effective. Here are some ideas that work:

- On the most basic level, hold **informational** meetings for nursing assistants. One finding from our research is that nursing assistants hear about state and federal policy changes, or funding cuts, and worry about them without really understanding them. Bring the nursing assistants together and **inform** them about what is going on. Make these meetings fun, by including recognition activities and announcements of events in nursing assistant's lives (like a new baby, or a child accepted to college). But also be sure that these meetings have **content.** Discuss plans for an upcoming state survey, or the impact of changes in your facility's administrative staff, or even what is going on with health care reform in Washington. Ask for their opinions, and really listen to them.

- Establish **problem-solving committees** that consist of representatives from the administration, the nursing staff, and the nursing assistants (as well as other relevant employees). Take a persistent problem — residents' laundry comes to mind — and put this interdisciplinary committee to work. Then use their suggestions. Use committees of nursing assistants for other activities, too, like planning an event (for example, Career Nurse Assistants Day).

- Allow the nursing assistants to help administration **set performance goals.** Rather than handing such goals down from on high, put together a group of nursing assistants to help you both decide on the goals, and also on how to implement them. For example, nursing assistants on a unit could tackle the problem of staff on the previous shift leaving too much work for the following shift, or of absenteeism. Of course, the nurses and administrators also take part in the process, but they use the nursing assistants' expertise to the greatest degree possible.

A Complete Overhaul

I noted earlier that it is also possible to take on job redesign in a big way. The Amherst Wilder Foundation in St. Paul, Minnesota, provides a good example of a serious attempt at job redesign. They felt their system of care was too fragmented and task-oriented. They were also worried about persistent staff dissatisfaction and turnover.

They responded by organizing staff into teams. Each team had a primary nurse and nursing assistants, who were assigned to a group of residents over the long term. These groups were also empowered to try to improve the quality of work and life in the facility. They did this, interestingly, in response to persistent worries about turnover and staff dissatisfaction.

The facility was divided into "nursing districts" of about twelve residents each. Small work groups were used to solve problems, including making suggestions about supplies and equipment, developing bath schedules, revising shift routines, and other areas. Nursing assistants operated on an equal footing with other staff in making decisions. In this facility, job satisfaction increased dramatically, and turnover dropped from a rate of 42% to less than 25%.

The key to the success of the Wilder Foundation's attempts at job redesign is to involve the nursing assistants as partners in improving the work life and quality of care in the facility. For job redesign to work, it must be participatory, and nursing assistants must feel that the changes are fair.

In discussing job redesign, I realize that I am proposing what for some facilities would be seen as a major change in the way that work is organized. However, even if you are not quite ready to take a major step, experimenting with some of the principles of job redesign can improve the work environment in your facility.

The payoffs are likely to be very great. Working as a team can be a powerful problem-solving tool, since nursing assistants know their **own** jobs — and, often, the residents — better than anyone else in the facility. And administrators who have tried opening up the decision-making process find that their own jobs become more enjoyable. An excited atmosphere develops in the facility, as new solutions are found for old problems. So by involving nursing assistants in decision-making, everyone benefits.

Another way to turn your nursing assistants into loyal allies is through training. Let's have a look now at how training, by involving your nursing assistants in a satisfying and empowering learning process, becomes a powerful retention tool.

CHAPTER EIGHT

Training: the Key to Retention

It is sometimes hard to talk to administrators about training. This is because many nursing homes feel they are already doing a good job preparing their staff for their work. A typical administrator might say: "Look — I am using a lot of resources to provide a good initial 75 hours of training. And then we train people on the job. How much more do we need to do?"

The answer is simple: A lot more. Because even if your nursing assistants are well trained in the **technical** aspects of resident care, you have done only half the job. This is what most nursing homes already do, and it is not helping them to retain their good nursing assistants.

Why is this? Because **nursing assistants often leave when they feel they do not have the skills and resources to handle the interpersonal aspects of resident care.** As we noted in Chapter 3, the job of nursing assistant requires relatively sophisticated psychosocial skills and understanding. To give an example, a nursing assistant may know all of the technical procedures for giving a resident a bath. But what does she do when the resident cries in fear of the shower, or begs to be left in bed, or strikes out at her while being washed?

So training in caregiving techniques is only the beginning. Equally important is continuing education about complex psychosocial issues. We can take as our motto another wise statement from Robert Desatnick: "People will do the right things, and do things right, if they are properly trained to do so."

Nursing assistants themselves feel the need for more education and training very keenly. In our focus groups, we have heard over and over: "We are the last ones to know anything around here." They feel that they are left out of the communication loop, that no one tells them anything.

I am devoting an entire chapter to training, because I think that enhanced training is the major retention tool that many nursing homes have **immediately** available to them. Many facilities feel an urgent need to begin to improve staff satisfaction and reduce turnover. Improving training is something you can do right away, and with very solid results.

Our research indicates the best weapon against turnover is **continuing education** that specifically deals with the **interpersonal aspects** of resident care. It is in ongoing training that the biggest gaps exist. Our research has found that inservice training for nursing assistants is haphazard at best. There is often no overall plan, and many staff are not aware of inservice opportunities.

This is particularly unfortunate, because training helps staff do their jobs better, and makes them enjoy their work more. However, it also serves another function. It says to the nursing assistant: "You are important! You mean a lot to us. It is worth it to us to invest in you." Our surveys show that nursing assistants who reported they had received special training in resident care issues that went beyond basic training were significantly less likely to be planning to leave.

It is worthwhile to emphasize a point made earlier:

> *We place nursing assistants in situations*
> *where unusually sophisticated interpersonal*
> *skills are needed, but we do not give them*
> *the resources to handle them.*

Consider what the typical nursing assistant, who is likely to have at most a high school education, and who has had 75 hours of technical training, is asked to do on a daily basis: negotiate conflict management, make ethical decisions, deal with bereavement, manage aggressive residents, and other complicated tasks. And they are asked to do these things **without any special training.** Frankly, we don't need research to tell us that training in how to handle complex psychosocial issues is necessary — we just need common sense!

Inservice Training on Specific Topics

Fortunately, there are a host of excellent training programs available today. You need to figure out what your needs are, and then pick among these. Here are a few good examples (for more examples, see Appendix 3):

1. *Values and Ethics for a Caring Staff in Nursing Homes*

Rosalie Kane and her colleagues developed this program to help nursing assistants recognize ethical issues and become comfortable in dealing with them. Ethical themes on which the program is based include fairness, respecting a residents' decision-making rights, and understanding values. The curriculum also looks at how these concepts apply to staff and residents, and covers the ethical obligations and responsibilities of nursing assistants. The curriculum provides an outline for ten sessions, and includes role-plays and case studies.

2. *Partners in Caregiving: Cooperative Communication Between Families and Nursing Homes*

Cornell University has recently developed this comprehensive training program to improve relationships between staff and family members. The training manual contains a number of different exercises that can be used in a facility, all of which take around one-half to one hour. The exercises explore such issues as how differences in values affect family-staff communication, the role of cultural and ethnic differences, ways of handling criticism and conflict, and other issues. The program also includes a parallel training for family members.

3. *Ensuring an Abuse-Free Environment: a Learning Program for Nursing Home Staff*

No one likes to talk about it, but there are times when nursing assistants act towards residents in ways they later regret. This outstanding program developed by Beth Hudson Keller at CARIE in Philadelphia trains nursing assistants in recognizing abusive behaviors. It also focuses heavily on prevention, by training staff to diffuse conflict before the situation gets out of hand. The units on how to respond to aggressive residents are especially helpful. Extensively tested in a number of nursing homes, and with an accompanying video, this training program goes far beyond its title in improving staff-resident relationships.

These are only three examples of the rich variety of new training materials that are available today. The point is this: Expand your horizons regarding what inservice training for nursing assistants can be. The days are long past when it was enough to focus only on the narrow, technical aspects of care. Keep your eyes open for new training materials that **really** help nursing assistants provide better quality care.

A Comprehensive Continuing Education Program

Another possibility is to provide regular, ongoing education in psychosocial resident care issues. To raise the status of nursing assistants and to help the long-term care industry meet the challenges of recruitment and retention, my colleagues and I developed **Nursing Assistant Monthly,** a multi-faceted training program for nursing assistants.

Each month enrolled facilities receive a training package, developed under the guidance of an editorial board of national experts, which includes a fully developed lesson-plan for the inservice coordinator, a guide to additional resources, and a quiz to measure learning and provide documentation that fulfills OBRA requirements for ongoing training of CNAs. The text for each month's topic is delivered to each CNA in the form of an attractive two-color newsletter that serves as their professional journal, building pride, confidence, and self-esteem. The newsletter includes an in-depth lead article, an interview with a national expert on the monthly topic, and a "Speaking from Experience" section that features advice and ideas from exceptional nursing assistants.

Each nursing assistant in a participating facility receives his or her own copy each month. This simple fact sends a powerful message to nursing assistants about their value as employees. Every profession needs to celebrate the hard work and value of its practitioners, and nursing assistants are no exception.

Some facilities have found the monthly training package so helpful that they organize their inservice training schedule around it.

Whether you decide to rely on occasional use of training programs on specific topics or to use a comprehensive continuing education program, the point is the same: **Start to make ongoing training work for you.** Just think about yourself. As a professional, you belong to associations, subscribe to journals, and talk to your peers about your work. This gives you a professional identity and a sense of purpose. Nursing assistants typically do not have anything like that. They as yet have no professional identity to call their own.

Meaningful training can help create such an identity, and can improve the self-esteem of your nursing assistants. It will also improve job satisfaction, and will slow down the revolving door.

CHAPTER NINE

The End — and a Beginning

Usually at this point in a report, the author gives a summary and some general conclusions. Frankly, I don't think that is necessary here. I want to use this last chapter to suggest a concrete way to get started improving your recruitment and retention situation.

A question you may be asking yourself is: What should I do now? Which of the options I've read about is the one for my facility? How should I prioritize my next steps? To set realistic goals that are appropriate for your nursing home, I suggest the following process.

Set aside time for a meeting exclusively devoted to recruitment and retention issues. If possible, try for a day-long session (a "retreat" outside the facility is a great idea). Put together the best group you can for this meeting: top administrative staff, nursing representatives, the inservice coordinator or personnel director, if you have one. Other participants might include members of a board of directors, and a local expert on gerontology or long-term care (perhaps from a nearby college or university). And, of course, include one or more experienced nursing assistants. The point is to get a wide range of perspectives represented.

Have the group members read this report, along with any other supporting information or data from your facility. (Here is a good chance to show off how carefully you calculate turnover rates!) Ask participants to come prepared to brainstorm about how to improve recruitment and retention in the facility.

To guide your discussion, use the list that appears in Appendix 1. In this list, I have noted all of the suggestions I made throughout this report. Ask the group to prioritize each item on this list.

The goal is obviously not to do everything; indeed, taking on too much is a good way to fail. It is fine to reject some of the options. But the group should try to be very clear **why** it has rejected an option. In my discussions with administrators, I have become accustomed to hearing "Yes, buts." Like, "Yes, that is a good idea, but it costs too much, takes too much time, etc." Using the group process, you can get beyond this "Yes, but" attitude by carefully specifying why an alternative is not right at the present time.

With the group's input, rate each option in the following way:

a) We are already doing this, and we are doing a good job.

b) We are already doing this, but we could improve what we are doing.

c) We aren't doing this, but we will begin right away.

d) We aren't doing this, but it's probably a good idea. We'll look into it.

e) We aren't doing this, and it's not right for us. (Be sure to specify the reasons why it isn't right.)

Once you get to the end of this list, you should have some very useful information. First, you may be surprised at everything you **are** doing right now. You will probably have the empowering feeling that you are on the right track in some areas. Second, you will have a clear set of priorities for your next steps. And finally, you will have ideas in reserve to try later. As you implement the new ideas, it will not take long to see a marked improvement in your recruitment and retention situation.

The Last Word

Since this report is all about how to improve the experience of nursing assistants, it seems right to give a nursing assistant the last word. One of the wisest people in the industry we have talked to over the years is Betty Brewer.

Mrs. Brewer has an unusual distinction: She was honored at the 1995 National Citizens' Coalition for Nursing Home Reform Convention as the longest-employed nursing assistant in the country, with 47 years of service! A living example of staff retention, she has been employed at Anna Marie of Aurora, in Aurora, Ohio, for the past 22 years.

As she puts it: "You have to like a place. I understand that a job's a job, but you have to like a place to want to stay on and do good work." Orient your efforts toward helping nursing assistants to "like the place" better, and you will be well on your way to shutting down the revolving door.

Recruitment and Retention: a Summary List

40 BRIGHT IDEAS

Measuring and Understanding Turnover

1. Calculate nursing assistant turnover rates every quarter.

2. Conduct exit interviews with departing staff.

3. Give current employees a job satisfaction survey.

4. Conduct focus groups with current employees.

Improving Recruitment

5. Recruit at local job fairs.

6. Hold a facility open house for potential employees.

7. Use local media for recruitment.

8. Provide bonuses to nursing assistants who recruit a new person.

9. Ask family members of residents to help recruit.

10. Get involved in a large-scale public awareness campaign.

11. Work with a local educational institution to begin a nursing assistant career training program.

12. Develop a more detailed screening interview for prospective nursing assistants.

13. Examine and revise your orientation program, to start new nursing assistants "on the right foot."

14. Give each new employee clear and detailed written materials at orientation.

15. Have the administrator personally recognize new staff during orientation.

16. Include some hands-on experience in the first day of orientation.

Staff Recognition

17. Increase public praise of nursing assistants. Implement the "praise at least one action a day" rule.

18. Write congratulatory letters to nursing assistants.

19. Create a supervisor evaluation-based recognition system for nursing assistants.

20. Create a peer evaluation-based recognition system for nursing assistants.

21. Celebrate Career Nurse Assistants Day.

22. Hold internal contests.

23. Establish employee of the month and unit of the month recognition programs.

24. Display letters from residents or family members.

25. Publish stories about nursing assistants in facility newsletters.

26. Place a recognition symbol on staff name badges.

27. Sponsor regular staff parties and outings.

28. Institute "Rookie of the Month" (or quarter) award.

29. Institute a "Supervisor of the Year" award, voted on by nursing assistants.

Retention Practices

30. Create a career ladder program for nursing assistants.

31. Consider permanent assignment of nursing assistants, instead of rotation.

32. Create a "buddy system" for nursing assistants.

33. Establish a nursing assistant support group.

34. Hold regular informational meetings for nursing assistants.

35. Establish problem-solving committees on specific issues.

36. Have nursing assistants participate in setting performance goals.

37. Carry out facility-wide job redesign.

Training

38. Institute regular inservice training on psychosocial and interpersonal aspects of resident care.

39. Review and obtain model inservice training programs on key issues.

40. Pursue comprehensive inservice education strategy.

A Bibliography

Chapter 2 — The Demographic Wake-up Call

Bayer, Ellen J., Stone, Robyn I. & Friedland, Robert B. (1993) "Developing a Caring and Effective Long-Term Care Workforce." Washington, D.C.: Project Hope: Center for Health Affairs (Final Report).

Breedlove, Janis. (June 1993) "The Career Door: Recruitment, Retention and Training of These Vital Workers Relies on One Thing: Motivation. Is It There?" *Nursing Homes*, pp. 8-9.

"Chronic Care Workers: Crisis Among Paid Caregivers of the Elderly." (1988) Washington, DC: Older Women's League.

Crowley, Carolyn Hughes. (December 1993) "The Human Factor: Unmasking Staff Potential." *Provider*, pp. 22-32.

Joint Commission on Accreditation of Healthcare Organizations, Chicago, Illinois. (1992) *Quality Improvement in Long Term Care.*

"Frontline Workers in Long-Term Care." (1994) *Generations: Journal of the American Society on Aging*, Vol. 17, No. 3.

Chapter 3 — Six Myths about Nursing Assistants

Bowers, Barbara & Becker, Marion. (1992) "Nurse's Aides in Nursing Homes: The Relationship Between Organization and Quality." *The Gerontologist*, Vol. 32, No. 3, pp. 360-366.

Brannon, Diane, Cohn, Margaret & Smyer, Michael A. (Spring 1990) "Caregiving as Work: How Nurse's Aides Rate It." *The Journal of Long-Term Care Administration*, pp. 10-14.

Brunk, Doug. (April 1995) "Show Some Respect: Nursing Assistants are a Vital Part of the Caregiving Team," *Contemporary Long-Term Care*, Vol. 18, No. 4, pp. 32-40.

Chappell, Neena L. & Novak, Mark. (1992) "The Role of Support in Alleviating Stress Among Nursing Assistants." *The Gerontologist*, Vol. 32, No. 3, pp. 351-359.

Crown, William H. (Fall 1994) "A National Profile of Home Care, Nursing Home, and Hospital Aides," *Generations*, Vol. 18, No. 3, pp. 29-33.

Diamond, Timothy. (1986) "Social Policy and Everyday Life in Nursing Homes: A Critical Ethnography." *Social Science and Medicine*, Vol. 23, No. 12, pp. 1287-1295.

Duncan, Marie T., and David L. Morgan. (1994) "Sharing the Caring: Family Caregivers' Views of Their Relationships with Nursing Home Staff." *The Gerontologist*, Vol. 34, No. 2, pp. 235-244.

Harvey Gittler. (September 6, 1993) "There's Skill in Unskilled Labor." *Industry Week*, p. 29.

Gubrium, Jaber. *Living and Dying in Murray Manor.* (1975) New York: St. Martin's Press.

Hare, Jan & Skinner, Denise. (Fall 1990) "The Relationship Between Work Environment and Burnout in Nursing Home Employees." *The Journal of Long Term Care Administration*, pp. 9-16.

Helmer, Theodore, Olson, Shirley, F. & Heim, Richard. (Summer 1995) "Strategies for Nurse Aide Job Satisfaction." *The Journal of Long-Term Care Administration*, pp. 10-14.

Hoffman, Richard. (April/May 1996) "Workforce Stability Starts with Respect." *Quality Care Advocate*, pp. 5-7

Monahan, Rita Short & McCarthy, Susanne. (1992) "Nursing Home Employment: The Nurse's Aide's Perspective." *Journal of Gerontological Nursing*, Vol. 18, No. 2, pp. 13-16.

National Citizens' Coalition for Nursing Home Reform. (1985 report) "A Consumer Perspective on Quality Care: the Resident's Point-of-view."

Porter, Lori J. (May 1992) "Preventing Job Burnout Enhances Nurse Assistant Satisfaction." *Provider*, pp. 59.

Tellis-Nayak, V. & Tellis-Nayak, Mary. (1989) "Quality of Care and the Burden of Two Cultures: When the World of the Nurse's Aide Enters the World of the Nursing Home." *The Gerontologist*, Vol. 29, No. 3, pp. 307-313.

Wilner, Mary Ann. (Fall 1994) "Working it Out: Support Groups for Nursing Assistants." *Generations*, Vol. 17, No. 3 pp. 39-40.

Chapter 4 — The Revolving Door (and Why It Turns)

Birkenstock, Marguerite. (July/August 1991) "From Turnover to Turnaround." *Geriatric Nursing*, pp. 194-196.

Bredenberg, Dave & Larsen, Cari. (November/December 1991) "Low Turnover Can Reap Great Rewards." *Nursing Homes*, pp. 5-7.

Bye, Margaret Gorely & Iannone, Joan. (July/August 1987) "Excellent Care-Givers (Nursing Assistants) of the Elderly: What Satisfies Them About Their Work." *Nursing Homes*, pp. 36-39.

Caudill, Marian E. & Patrick, Maxine. (Winter 1991-92) "Turnover Among Nursing Assistants: Why They Leave and Why They Stay." *The Journal of Long-Term Care Administration*, pp. 29-32.

Feldman, Penny Hollander. (February 1989) "The Ford Home Care Project: Reducing Turnover Among Paraprofessionals." *Caring*, pp. 28-29.

Garland, Neal T., Oyabu, Naoko & Gipson, Genevieve, A. (1989) "Job Satisfaction Among Nurse Assistants Employed in Nursing Homes: An Analysis of Selected Job Characteristics." *Journal of Aging Studies*, Vol. 3, No. 4, pp. 369-383.

Garland, T. Neal, Oyabu, Naoko & Gipson, Genevieve A. (Winter 1988) "Stayers and Leavers: A Comparison of Nurse Assistants Employed in Nursing Homes." *The Journal of Long Term Care Administration*, pp. 23-29.

Kruzich, Jean M., Clinton, Jacqueline F. & Kelbert, Sheryl T. (1992) "Personal and Environmental Influences on Nursing Home Satisfaction." *The Gerontologist*, Vol. 32, No. 3, pp. 342-350.

Marvin, Bill. (1994) *From Turnover to Teamwork: How to Build and Retain a Customer-oriented Foodservice Staff*. John Wiley & Sons.

Wagnild, Gail & Manning, Roger W. (Summer 1986) "The High-Turnover Profile: Screening and Selecting Applicants for Nurse's Aide." *The Journal of Long-Term Care Administration*, pp. 2-4.

Waxman, Howard M., Carner, Erwin A. & Berkenstock, Gale. (1984) "Job Turnover and Job Satisfaction Among Nursing Home Aides." *The Gerontologist*, Vol. 24, No. 5, pp. 503-509.

Winger, Jean Merhige & Smythe-Staruch, Kathleen. (1986) "Your Patient is Older: What Leads to Job Satisfaction?" *Journal of Gerontological Nursing*, Vol. 12, No. 1, pp. 31-35.

Chapter 5 — Recruiting for Excellence

Buss, Dale D. (September 1994) "As the Staff Turns." *Contemporary Long-Term Care.* pp. 61-64.

Everett, Harvey A. (December 1994) "Starting Out on the Right Foot." *Residential Living,* pp 51-52.

"Fifteen Bright Ideas in Recruitment, Training, and Management." (Fall 1994) *Human Resources and Aging,* (see Appendix 3).

Levinsion, Jay Conrad. (1989) *Guerrilla Marketing Attack.* Boston: Houghton Mifflin.

Thomas, Mark & Brull, Harry. (November 1993) "Tests Improve Hiring Decisions at Franciscan." *Personnel Journal,* pp. 89-92.

Chapter 6 — Recognizing Real Worth

Desatnick, Robert L. (1990) *Keep the Customer!* Boston: Houghton Mifflin.

Chapter 7 — Three "Best Practices" to Retain Nursing Assistants

Brannon, Diane, Smyer, Michael A., Cohn, Margaret D., Borchardt, Lawrence, Landry, Julie A., Jay, Gina M., Garfein, Adam J., Malonebeach, Eileen & Walls, Carla. (1988) "A Job Diagnostic Survey of Nursing Home Caregivers: Implications for Job Redesign." *The Gerontologist,* Vol. 28, No. 2, pp. 246-252.

Greater New York Hospital Foundation, Inc. (1992) Project Linc: Ladders in Nursing Careers (annual report).

Hegland, Anne. (September 1990) "Upgrading Care and Improving Retention: Genesis Offers Aides, Nurses Special Incentives." *Contemporary Long-Term Care.*

Kruzich, Jean M. (1995) "Empowering Organizational Contexts: Patterns and Predictors of Perceived Decision-Making Influence Among Staff in Nursing Homes." *The Gerontologist*, Vol. 35, No. 2, pp. 207-216.

McDonald, Carolyn A. (Winter 1991-1992) "Career Ladder: Tool for Recruitment, Retention, and Recognition." *The Journal of Long-Term Care Administration*, pp. 6-7.

Kari, Nancy & Michels, Peg. (February 1991) "The Lazarus Project: The Politics of Empowerment." *The American Journal of Occupational Therapy*, pp. 719-725.

Patchner, Michael A. & Patchner, Lisa S. (June 1993) "Essential Staffing for Improved Nursing Home Care: The Permanent Assignment Model." *Nursing Homes.* pp. 37-39.

Teresi, Jeanne, Holmes, Douglas, Benenson, Esther, Monaco, Charlene, Barrett, Virginia, Ramirez, Mildred & Koren, Mary Jane. (1993) "A Primary Care Nursing Model in Long-Term Care Facilities: Evaluation of Impact on Affect, Behavior, and Socialization." *The Gerontologist*, Vol. 33, No. 5, pp. 667-674.

Wilner, Mary Ann. (Fall 1994) "Working it Out: Support Groups for Nursing Assistants." *Generations*, Vol. 17, No. 3 pp. 39-40.

Chapter 8 — Training: the Key to Retention

Burgio, Louis, D. & Burgio, Kathryn L. (1990) "Institutional Staff Training and Management: A Review of the Literature and a Model for Geriatric, Long-term Care Facilities." *International Journal Aging and Human Development*, Vol. 30, No. 4, pp. 287-302.

Burgio, Louis D. & Scilley, Kay. (1994) "Caregiver Performance in the Nursing Home: The Use of Staff Training and Management Procedures." *Seminars in Speech and Language*, Vol. 15, No. 4, pp. 313-322.

Ernst, Nora S. & West, Helen L. (1983) *Nursing Home Staff Development: A Guide for Inservice Programs.* New York: Springer Publishing Company.

Filinson, Rachel. (1994) "An Evaluation of a Gerontological Training Program for Nursing Assistants." *The Gerontologist,* Vol. 34, No. 6, pp. 839-843.

Heiselman, Terry & Noelker, Linda S. (1991) "Enhancing Mutual Respect Among Nursing Assistants, Residents, and Residents' Families." *The Gerontologist,* Vol. 31, No. 4, pp. 552-555.

Hoffman, Richard. (May 1996) "Is This Any Way to Run an Airline? Top Companies' Lessons for Long-term Care Training." *Nursing Homes,* pp. 10-12.

Hoffman, Richard. (November 1995) "Training Nursing Assistants Translates into Better Care." *The Brown University Long-Term Care Quality Letter,* Vol. 7, No. 21. p. 6.

Maas, Meridean, Buckwalter, Kathleen Coen, Swansin, Elizabeth & Mobily, Paula. (Spring 1994) "Training Key to Job Satisfaction." *Long-Term Care Administration,* Vol. 11, No. 1, pp. 23-26.

Peck, Richard L. (June 1995) "New Concepts in Recruitment and Retention: an Interview with Karl Pillemer, Ph.D." *Nursing Homes,* pp. 8-12.

Smyer, Michael, Brannon, Diane & Cohn, Margaret. (1992) "Improving Nursing Home Care Through Training and Job Redesign." *The Gerontologist,* Vol. 32, No. 3, pp. 327-333.

Turkington, Carol. (September/October 1992) "Training for Nurse Assistants: What's Available." *Nursing Homes,* pp. 23-26.

Whittier, Tim. (August 1995) "Finding and Keeping Good Direct Care Staff" *Provider,* pp. 42-43.

A Resource Guide

GENERAL RESOURCES

- A good resource is a special issue of the journal *Generations* (Vol. 18, Fall 1994), published by the American Society on Aging. This issue, titled "Front-Line Workers in Long-Term Care," looks at the problems such workers encounter, as well as proposing ways that long-term care institutions can respond to these workers' needs. Some of the articles deal with home health workers, which provides an interesting contrast to those about nursing homes. To order this issue, contact:

      Generations
      American Society on Aging
      833 Market Street, Room 511
      San Francisco, CA 94103-1824
      (415) 974-9600

- Another excellent source of information is the **National Eldercare Institute on Human Resources,** run by the Brookdale Center on Aging. They publish the newsletter *Human Resources & Aging,* which covers resources and practices for recruitment, training, and management/supervision of staff. Two recent issues are particularly relevant: the Fall, 1994 issue presents "Fifteen

Bright Ideas in Recruitment, Training, and Management," and the Summer, 1994 issue highlights winners of a "Best Practice" competition. In addition, they have a variety of information packets and lists of film resources. They also maintain files of written information so that inquiries can be referred to appropriate other agencies. You can contact the center at the following address:

> National Eldercare Institute on Human Resources
> Brookdale Center on Aging
> 425 East 25th Street
> New York, NY 10010
> (212) 481-4350

- *Provider* magazine, published by the American Health Care Association, frequently has articles on nursing assistant recruitment and retention. The December, 1993, issue's lead article called "The Human Factor: Unmasking Staff Potential" is a must-read.

- A recent report from Project Hope is very useful. The report, **"Developing a Caring and Effective Long-Term Care Workforce"** by Ellen Bayer, Robyn Stone, and Robert Friedland, can be requested from:

> Project Hope
> Center for Health Affairs
> 7500 Old Georgetown Road, Suite 600
> Bethesda, MD 20814-6133
> (301) 656-7401

STAFF SCREENING

- Franciscan Health System of Dayton, OH, has developed a **Nursing Assistant Test Battery,** consisting of three separate tests. They report a major drop in turnover using these tests to help select nursing assistants. For more information, contact Franciscan at (513) 229-6527.

  An article on the program is also available: "Tests Improve Hiring Decisions at Franciscan," by Mark Thomas and Harry Brull, *Personnel Journal,* November 1993, pp. 89-92.

CAREER LADDER PROGRAMS

- The **"Geriatric Nursing Assistant Specialist Program"** aims to upgrade the skills and enhance the self-esteem of nursing assistants. Students complete a training program that covers a number of aspects of resident care. Information is available from:

  > Educational Pathways, Inc.
  > 916 Shaker Road, #336
  > Longmeadow, MA 01106
  > (413) 783-0291

- For a program that helps nursing assistants obtain an LPN or RN degree, information is available from **Project LINC,** which has an impressive track record in this area. Contact:

  > Peggy McNally-Temme
  > Greater New York Hospital Foundation, Inc.
  > 555 West 57th Street, Room 1500
  > New York, NY 10019
  > (212) 246-7100

STAFF RECOGNITION

- If you are interested in **Career Nurse Assistants Day**, a detailed planning guide and other information are available from:
    Genevieve Gipson
    Career Nurse Assistants Program, Inc.
    3577 Easton Road
    Norton, OH 44203-5661

PUBLIC AWARENESS CAMPAIGNS

- For information about Massachusetts' experience with public awareness campaigns to recruit nursing assistants, contact Petra Langer, **Massachusetts Extended Care Federation** (617) 558-0202.

SUPPORT GROUPS FOR NURSING ASSISTANTS

- A video entitled **"Working it Out: Support Groups for Nursing Aides,"** and an accompanying training manual are available from Terra Nova Films at 800-779-8491. For additional information about this program, contact:
    Mary Ann Wilner, Ph.D.
    387 Sixth Street
    Brooklyn, NY 11215
    (718) 965-1337

JOB TRAINING PROGRAMS

- Programs that train people for careers as paraprofessionals in long-term care are profiled in the Fall, 1994 issue of *Human Resources and Aging*, available from the Brookdale Center on Aging, (212) 481-4350.

SELECTED TRAINING MATERIALS

There are a variety of training materials now available on the psychosocial aspects of nursing home care. The programs noted in the report are as follows:

- **Nursing Assistant Monthly**
  The result of more than ten years of research into the lives of nursing assistants by Dr. Karl Pillemer of Cornell University, this ongoing training program is designed to address the critical interpersonal and psychosocial aspects of caregiving.

  Each month's training package, developed under the guidance of an editorial board of national experts, includes a fully developed lesson-plan for the inservice coordinator, a guide to additional resources, and a quiz to measure learning and provide documentation that fulfills OBRA requirements for ongoing training of CNAs. The text for each month's topic is delivered to each CNA in the form of an attractive newsletter that serves as their professional journal, building pride, confidence, and self-esteem.

  Past issues have focused on topics such as Problem Behaviors in Dementia, Dealing with Death on the Job, Managing Aggressive Residents, Effective Communication Skills, Preventing Back Injuries, and Balancing Work and Family. For more information, contact:
  Nursing Assistant Monthly
  Frontline Publishing Corp.
  17 Herbert St., PO Box 441002
  Somerville, MA 02144
  Toll-free: 1-800-348-0605

- **Values and Ethics for a Caring Staff in Nursing Homes**
  Rosalie Kane, DSW
  National LTC Resource Center
  School of Public Health
  University of Minnesota
  Minneapolis, MN 55455
  (612) 624-6669

- **AGE Institute**
  AGE Institute is a non-profit organization which offers professional development and inservice programs to health care professionals of all levels and disciplines. Their programs range from one-hour inservice programs to one- and two-day seminars. They have also been pioneers in the important area of work-readiness, including the adult literacy program, Workplace Instruction Now, or WIN. This program was developed to provide on-site delivery of a healthcare-based literacy program. The 12-week, 48-hour program is designed for entry and service level staff. The WIN pilot program resulted in improvement of 1 to 1.5 grade levels in six academic categories. For information contact:
  Angela D. Stoops, BS, RN
  Director of Educational Services
  AGE Institute
  The Professional Arts Bldg.
  25 Penncraft Ave.
  Chambersburg, PA 17201
  (717) 263-7766

- **Ensuring an Abuse-Free Environment**
    Beth Hudson Keller
    CARIE
    1315 Walnut Street, Suite 1000
    Philadelphia, PA 19107
    (215) 545-5728

- **Partners in Caregiving**
    Partners in Caregiving consists of two parallel workshop series, one for family members and one for nursing home staff. The staff workshop is structured as an inservice day, and the family program includes three two-hour sessions. Topics covered include advanced listening skills, understanding value differences, and handling blame, criticism, and conflict. The project ends with a combined session with families, staff, and facility administrative staff. For information contact:
    Human Development and Family Studies, MVR Hall
    Cornell University
    Ithaca, NY 14850
    (607) 255-8086